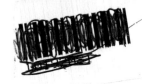
LEANER FITTER STRONGER

Get the body you want with our *amazing meals* & *smart workouts*

We would like to dedicate this book to the entirety of the LDNMFamily who have been there since the beginning, and to those who have joined our journey along the way – offering their support and encouragement. Your loyalty has been invaluable and provides the motivation for us to keep making key changes in the fitness industry; from exclusive and unattainable, to inclusive, realistic, fun, effective and healthy!

10 9 8 7 6 5 4 3 2 1

Vermilion, an imprint of Ebury Publishing,
20 Vauxhall Bridge Road,
London, SW1V 2SA

Vermilion is part of the Penguin Random House group of companies whose addresses can be found at global.penguinrandomhouse.com

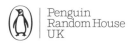

Penguin
Random House
UK

Text © Lloyd Bridger, Max Bridger, James Exton and Tom Exton 2017
Photography © Howard Shooter 2017: pages 4–5, 8 (Tom and James), 16, 19, 31–2, 46–152, 266–7 / © Malcolm Griffiths 2017: pages 8 (Max and Lloyd), 12, 15, 163–254

Lloyd Bridger, Max Bridger, James Exton and Tom Exton have asserted their right to be identified as the authors of this Work in accordance with the Copyright, Designs and Patents Act 1988

Design: Maru Studio
Food styling: Moo Jevons

First published by Vermilion in 2017

www.penguin.co.uk

A CIP catalogue record for this book is available from the British Library

ISBN: 9781785040887

Printed and bound in Italy by Printer Trento

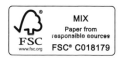

MIX
Paper from
responsible sources
FSC® C018179
www.fsc.org

Penguin Random House is committed to a sustainable future for our business, our readers and our planet. This book is made from Forest Stewardship Council® certified paper.

The information in this book has been compiled by way of general guidance in relation to the specific subjects addressed, but it is not a substitute and not to be relied on for medical, healthcare, pharmaceutical or other professional advice on specific circumstances and in specific locations. Please consult your GP before changing, stopping or starting any medical treatment. So far as the authors are aware the information given is correct and up to date as at January 2017. Practice, laws and regulations all change, and the reader should obtain up to date professional advice on any such issue. The author and the publishers disclaim, as far as the law allows, any liability arising directly or indirectly from the use or misuse of the information contained in this book.

LEANER FITTER STRONGER

Get the body you want
with our *amazing meals*
& *smart workouts*

THE EXTON TWINS & BRIDGER BROTHERS – *Founders of* **LDNM**®

Vermilion
LONDON

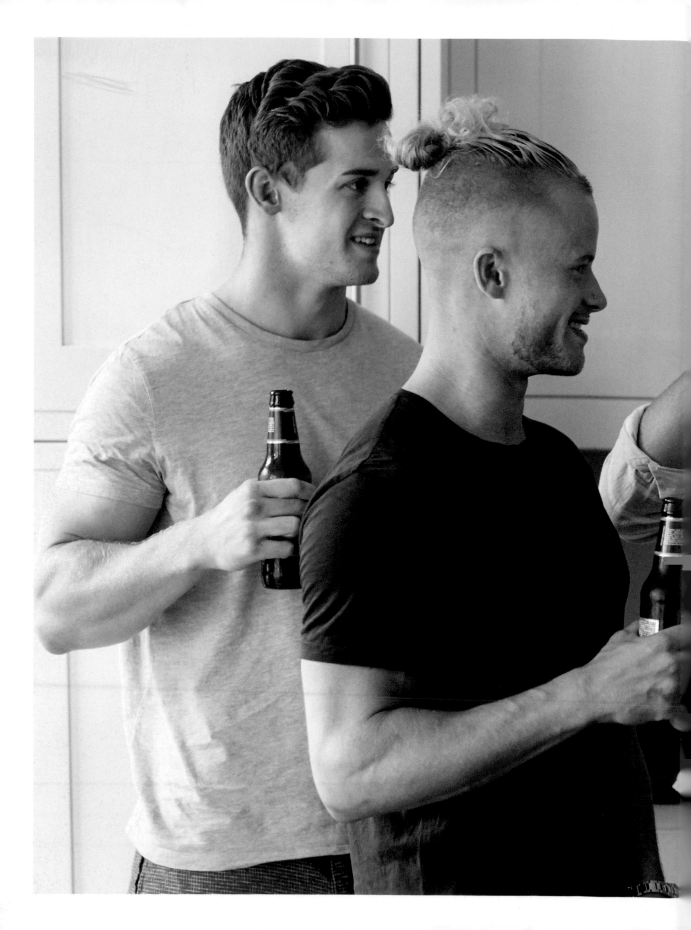

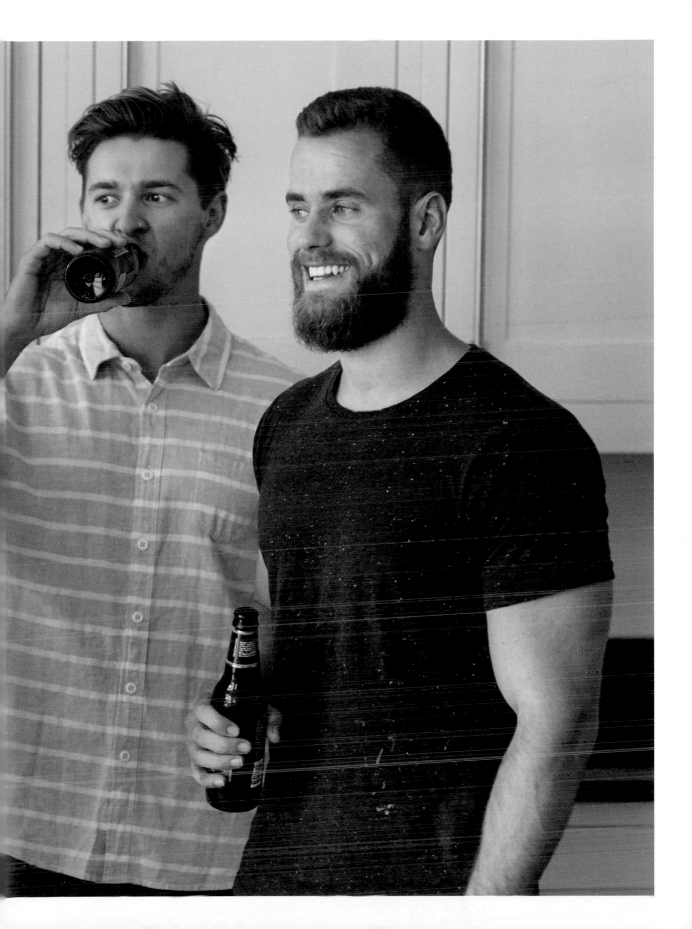

CONTENTS

WELCOME   9

LDNM – who we are   10
    Lloyd   12
    Max   14
    Tom   16
    James   18
How to use this book   20

GETTING STARTED   21

Measuring your progress   22
Weight loss   23
Muscle building   26
Set your goal   27
Keywords, acronyms and
    buzzwords decoded   28
Success at any size   30

LEANER   33

Track your week   34
'Good' vs 'bad' foods   35
Supplements   36
Flexible dieting   39
Myth busting   39
Stocking up   43
Breakfast   45
Lunch   61
Dinner   81
Snacks & on the go   117
The sweet stuff   125
4-ingredient heroes   143

FITTER 153

|||||||||||||||||||||||||||||||||||||||

Myth busting	154
High-Intensity Interval Training (HIIT)	156
Tabata circuits	162
Gym-free workouts	182
Buddy training	195
Gym training	202
Stretches	244

STRONGER   255

|||||||||||||||||||||||||||||||||||||||

Willpower vs perseverance	256
Marginal gains	257
Keeping up motivation	258
Checking in with your goals	260
Plateaus	261
Fitting fitness into work and social life	262
Visualisation	264
Negative self-talk	265
Tracking your progress	267

Index	274
Results	283
Acknowledgements	286

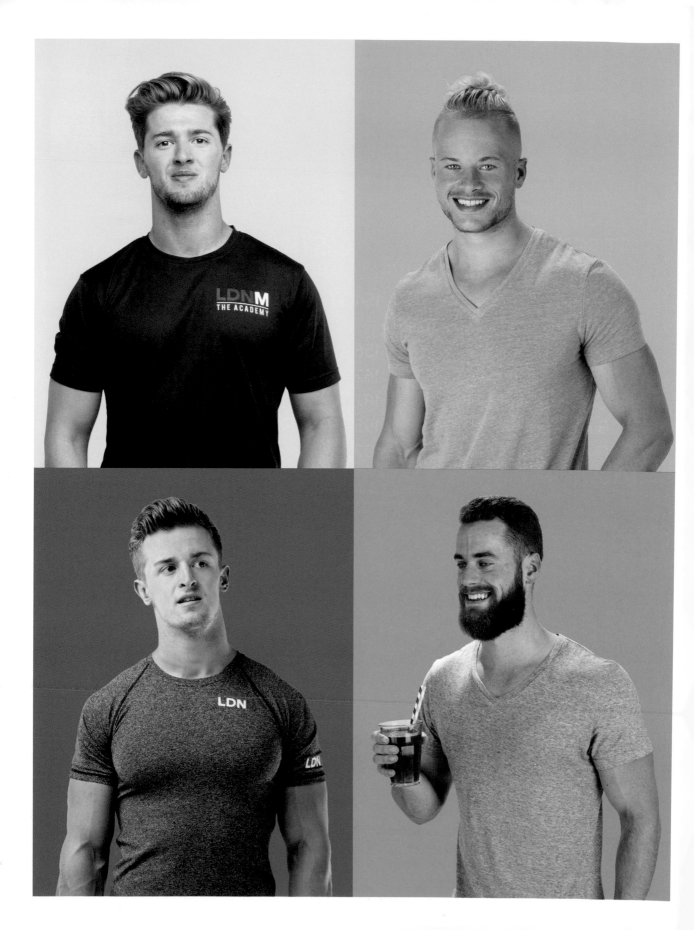

Welcome

||||||||||||||||||||||||||||||||||||||||||||||||||||||||||||||||||||

Hey – welcome! We're so pleased you're here :-)

In your hands you have the tools to reveal a happier and healthier You, in other words, You, but Leaner, Fitter and Stronger. There's no 'New You' philosophy in these pages – we're pretty certain that you're already pretty good as you are. But all of us at some point have decided to make a change – whether you have been studying too hard and want to exercise your bodies as well as your minds, maybe you're feeling sluggish and want to kick-start your system, maybe you're recovering from an operation, or just want to feel better in your clothes. Whatever your reason, and whatever your mission, you can be sure of one thing: we'll be with you every step of the way.

We promise that this book is BS-free. There are no pie-in-the-sky promises here. We want the changes that you make to be long-lasting, and definitely not the kind of quick fixes that lead you down the path of yo-yo dieting. We want to help you develop a new lifestyle that is fun, effective, good value and sustainable. None of us can stand fitness idols and celebrities who promote the latest fad without solid evidence backing their statements. Fitness can be simple, and a beneficial addition to your lifestyle – mentally, physically and aesthetically – and this book will arm you with the tools to achieve this.

LDNM – who we are

||||||||||||||||||||||||||||||||||||||||||||||||||||||||||||||||||||||||||||||||||||||||||||||||||||||||||||

LDNM was created in 2013 as an interactive platform for us four guys – James, Tom, Lloyd and Max – to answer the ever-increasing number of questions we were receiving regarding our training and nutrition, health and fitness.

We started out working as lifeguards at Hampton Open Air Pool, our local leisure centre, and trained together at the humble poolside gym within the facility. We made a point of doing so steroid free, and did our best to help colleagues and other gym members reach their fitness goals.

We soon began to grow a small local following, and a reputation in the local area among younger guys and girls for delivering results. At this point the fifth member of Team LDNM approached us with the idea to create a website and social media platform to answer questions, and to provide content on realistic training and nutrition to build muscle or lose fat. We agreed, seeing it as a hobby and even a time saver, but we never saw it snowballing into the movement and brand it has become today!

Online engagement was strong from the outset, and incredibly exciting for us. After being burned by supplement companies and fitness models – wasting our pay cheques on supplements promising (and costing) the world – we set out to tell it like it is to normal people. Unsurprisingly we experienced a lot of friction from the fitness industry, which had been conning people unchallenged for too long, with supplement companies offering us sponsorships and individuals with more followers on social media trying to stamp us out. However, we kept true to our mission to expose the clouded industry of fitness, and to show people how they can get leaner, fitter and stronger without negatively affecting their bank balance and quality of life! Thankfully, people liked our message, and the LDNM movement is going from strength to strength.

We have come a long way since 2013, and built our following to over 400,000 people across Twitter, Instagram and Facebook. It's both our aim and our pleasure to maintain a personal rapport with our loyal and new followers alike!

Our LDNM transformation guides, which cover training, nutrition, supplements and lifestyle for men and women, have gone from simple Word documents to industry-leading guides in quality and quantity of information and support. These guides have allowed hundreds of thousands of normal people like ourselves, people with busy work, school and social lives, to progress their fitness goals sustainably, and we are proud of each and every success story, no matter how small.

We've also launched a successful line of apparel for training and outerwear, as well as developing effective, good-quality supplements that are available for a fair price. The LDNM Academy was developed to better the industry standard of teaching, as we felt that some operators were damaging their clients' health, bank balance and attitude towards health and fitness. The Academy has come on leaps and bounds since it was started in 2015: personal training courses, nutrition coaching courses and social media events across London have all been sell outs.

Our website and social media channels are packed full of training, nutrition and lifestyle-based content (you can find us at www.ldnmuscle.com). We aim to show people how to achieve genuine balance and make fitness and nutrition an enjoyable and valuable part of their lives. Getting leaner, fitter and stronger should not be to the detriment of the lifestyle you enjoy.

We have invested time, energy and passion into LDNM from the moment it started. We wanted to create – and we believe we have created – a safe, sustainable and realistic approach to health and fitness, for anyone of any size or background. We wouldn't be where we are today without the unprecedented level of support from you and everyone else reading this right now, and we are so truly grateful for it. We all want to say a huge personal thank you from all of us to all of you.

" Success
can come
at any size "

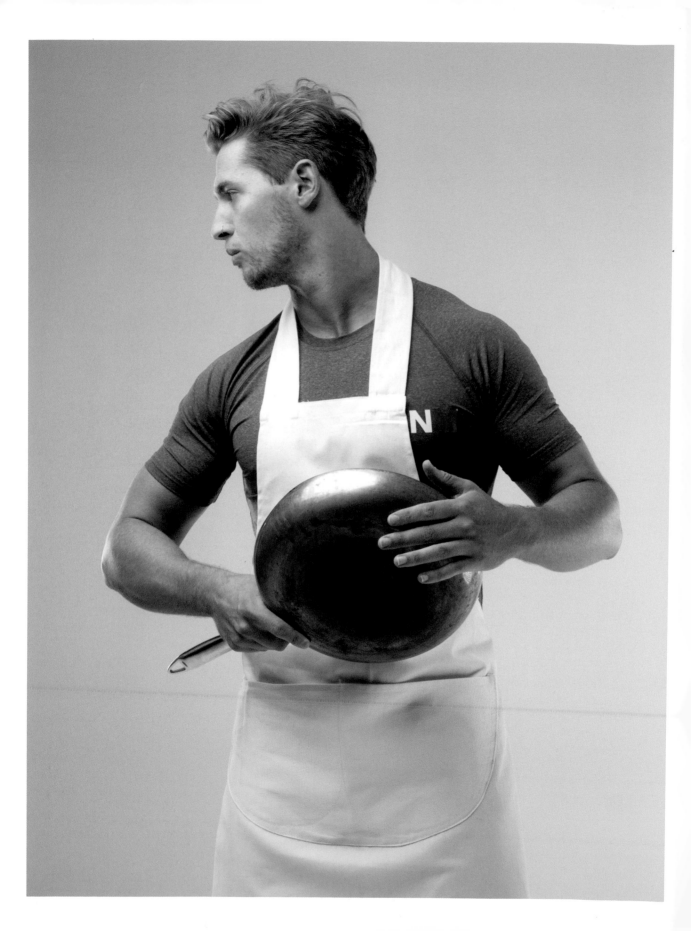

Lloyd

||||||||||||||||||||||||||||||||||||||||||||||||||||||||||||||||||||||||||||||||||||||||||||||||||||||

I'm the oldest of three – Max, Lilly and me – and we've always been competitive, whether it was eating, school or sport. Our parents were keen to channel this competitiveness in a more productive way, each finding time between their two jobs to ferry us to any sport club within a five-mile radius – everything from gymnastics (you could never tell now) to kayaking. Triathlon turned out to be the sport I was least bad at (it's easier to be bad at three sports than it is one), and I spent most of my teenage years doing this, as well as playing football and riding bikes.

I left home to read chemistry at the University of Bristol, only to find that there was no university triathlon club. When a second-year student told me that rowing was the hardest thing he had ever done, I decided that sounded like the sport for me. It was here that my crewmate and good friend Pablo introduced me to weights, or 'sculpting', as he liked to call it, and I haven't looked back. Being naturally very slight, those first few months of muscle gain felt great and I caught the lifting bug. I didn't have any particular physique in mind, I just wanted to be bigger than the 10-stone triathlete I was! Over my three years at uni the majority of my time was dedicated to rowing and lifting, training anywhere between eight and twelve times a week, and my studies fitted around this.

We won some big races and I built some muscle, but ended up leaving with a 2:2 and no idea of the direction I was going to take next. In my gap year at Hampton Pool I worked and trained with Max, James and Tom while weighing up my options as a graduate in the middle of the recession. It was here I decided to pursue my lifelong ambition of becoming a Royal Marines Officer, something I didn't undertake lightly.

Only taking one batch of around 50 officers each year, it was always going to be a tough process and in 2012 I fell just short at the Admiralty Interview Board; they suggested I retry the next year. It was this year that James, Tom, Max and I decided to start LDNM.

In 2013 I attempted to pass the AIB for the Royal Marines for the second time and I was offered a place for the 2013 intake. Taking up this place would have meant giving up LDNM as the two years of officer training would have taken up all of my time. I decided to take the biggest risk of my life and turn down my place in order to pursue LDNM, hoping it was the right thing to do.

Fast forward three years and LDNM has become a well-known, reputable brand with over 50,000 customers, providing realistic information that helps to change people's lives. There has been a lot of blood, sweat and tears along the way, but it has definitely been worth it.

Working at LDNM is great, but at times unpredictable as my schedule can change at short notice. Mixing work with training while seeing my friends regularly for a social drink or two, means I often end up grabbing food on the go. Contrary to what you might believe – and what you've been told – you can do all of this and stay in great shape; you can enjoy your food (actual food, not just salads) and a social life and still get the physique you want. All will be explained later in the book!

Max

||||||||||||||||||||||||||||||||||||||||||||||||||||||||||||||||||||||||||||||||||||||||||||||||||||||

I'm a normal 25-year-old guy who loves a drink, a meal out, a holiday (or two) and spending time with my family and friends. I've always been involved in sports, competing in triathlon, cycling and football. Unfortunately, two to five hours of exercise a day caught up with me, leaving me with a chronic hip injury, which I've managed since I was 16.

It was then I started work at my local leisure centre, where my brother Lloyd and the Exton twins introduced me to weight training. Lifting replaced sports for me and at first it was as much about vanity as it was about fitness: I wanted to look good, plain and simple!

In my naïve enthusiasm, I wasted money on supplements that promised me a Hollywood-style physique. I also wasted my time and risked my health with ridiculous eating and training styles. At one point I would not eat any carbohydrates after midday as the fitness media had demonised carbohydrates so much that I thought this was the answer. In addition to this I would do one to two sessions of cardio a day in an attempt to burn fat. This was completely unsustainable and luckily I realised this after I rebounded – putting on weight quickly – and becoming ill after a lads' holiday in Magaluf.

I've since completed a degree in geography (BSc) at the University of Birmingham while co-running LDNM. During this time I blogged about balancing university life with training and affordable nutrition, as well as co-writing the LDNM Guides. Finding time for the gym became relatively hard in my second and third years, but planning ahead of time and using exercise as my breaks and downtime resolved this more often than not.

Since I graduated in 2014 I have built a career as a personal trainer while also running LDNM full-time. My working week can be between 40 and 70 hours and is a constantly changing mix of clients and LDNM duties. This makes training and nutrition an issue, but planning my days as realistically as possible and training before breakfast means I rarely stop progressing towards my goals!

I absolutely love what I do, helping my clients reach their goals and couldn't think of another job I would rather take on.

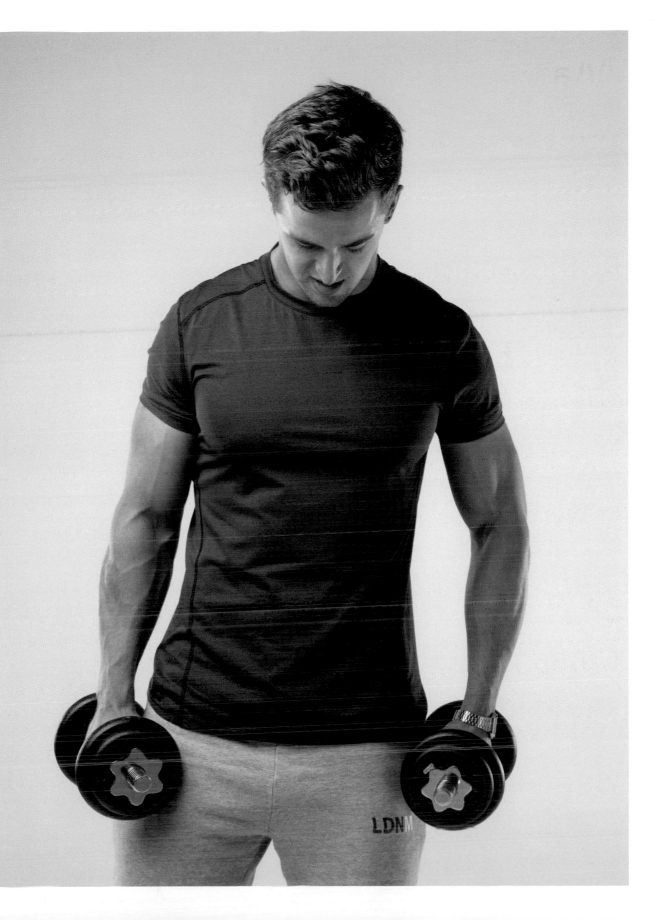

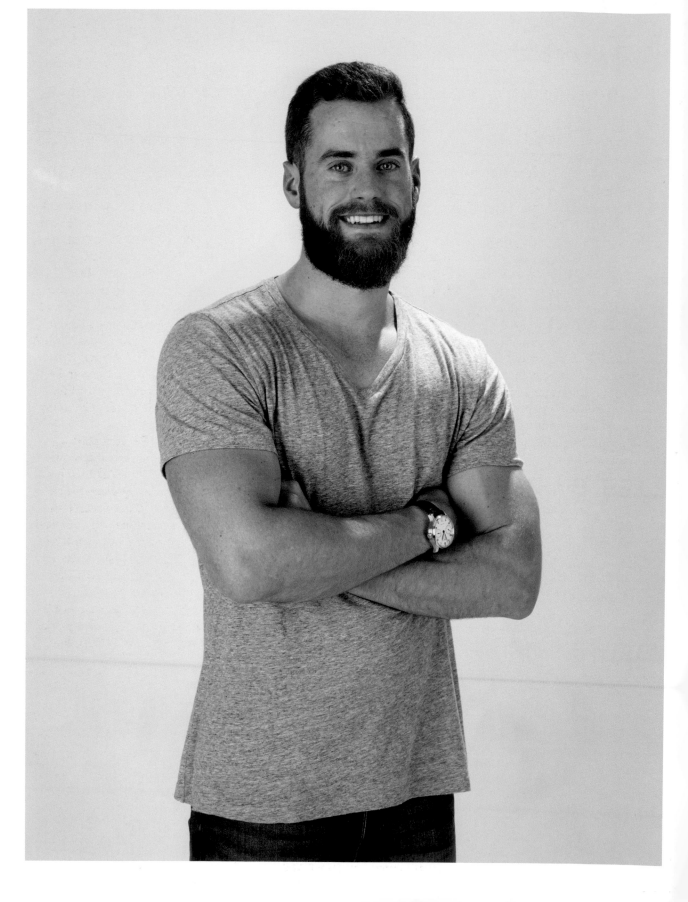

Tom

||||||||||||||||||||||||||||||||||||||||||||||||||||||||||||||||||||||||||||||||||||||||||||

As a young chap, I used to do pretty much every sport under the sun alongside my twin: swimming, cross-country, tennis, football, triathlon – you name it. I think this was partly because James and I had far too much energy, and partly our parents' way of getting us tired to give them some peace and quiet.

Fast forward a few years and I began 'training' in the gym while I was at university. By then, I had jacked in my sporting exploits in favour of lie-ins and going out. I put 'training' in inverted commas, because it was nothing more than cluelessly snatching at heavy things sporadically in the gym whenever I had a few minutes between lectures and daytime TV. This went on for about a year, until I actually started looking into what I was doing, and – most importantly – what I was eating. I've been 'properly' training now for about six years and am still learning every day.

My student days are long gone. These days I work full time, on top of my role with LDNM. Finding the time is often an issue; working for a bank in the City for the past five years, with an inhumane commute and running a business or two on the side – it's tough sometimes to squeeze that session in. Even if I can find a small window, I sometimes have to dig deep and ask if I can be bothered. Ultimately, though, I ensure I find time as I always feel so much better for it. Even if it's just 20–30 minutes – I'll make it happen. I'll just sacrifice a bit of dubious television in the evening. Something I can live with.

Currently I work out around five times a week. A lot of these sessions will be a 'lunchtime' 25–35 minute job in the city. I find it more than enough time for the smaller muscle groups if you keep it intense. This said – legs are often Saturdays, and chest sometimes finds its way into a Sunday.

I always get asked what my diet is like. Answer? By no means perfect. I try to follow my macros as best as I can, but given my work and social life, I often fail to prepare meals (shock horror). When this happens I make do with what I can find in 'express' supermarkets near the office. Not ideal, but I feel compromise can be found occasionally without ruining your life. I make sure I've always got healthy snacks in my desk for emergencies.

The main driving force at the very start of my 'training' was a mixture of curiosity, a touch of boredom and a desire to fill my T-shirt out a tad. Gradually, though, fitness developed into a routine and a way of life, and now I can't see myself ever not being active in one form or other.

My motivation? It may seem shallow but I'm going to admit it: a large part is just wanting look as good as I can. I'm sure many will echo this sentiment, possibly, just maybe not out loud… That said, being healthy and fit is just as important to me – there's no point looking great if underneath you're unhealthy, feel awful and can't run for a bus.

James

I've always been active. When I wasn't wrestling with my twin brother Tom, I'd be found playing a host of sports: football, rugby, tennis, swimming, triathlon.

But as education begun to take hold, with GCSEs and A-Levels, time became more limited, I was unable to commit to the training timetables required for competitive-level sports without affecting my studies. Sport became a hobby.

I studied law at Nottingham University, before being awarded a scholarship to Nottingham Law School to complete the BVC (Bar Vocational Course) to enable me to qualify as a barrister. It was during my first year at uni that I discovered the gym. Seeing other guys on campus with their tops off in summer and grabbing all the attention, made me realise, for the first time ever, that I wanted to be in 'good shape'. By this I mean lean with a six pack. At the time I saw myself more as a skinny sausage-shaped body! I started going to the gym a couple of times a week with a few uni friends, and became more and more motivated to change the way I looked. I began to read up about training and nutrition, and started to radically change the way I looked.

When I came home for half-term, Tom said 'How the hell did you do that?' The progress was clear, and he was absolutely livid, so much so he got the bit between his teeth and started training with me and continued it back at his uni. There is nothing to compete with the rivalry between twins!

Following university and law school I was formally called to the bar and went to work in Oxford Street for a criminal law firm. Despite long hours and long commutes, I always made time for the gym. It was a good stress-release and I always found a way to effectively manage the work–play balance.

As criminal law is a predominantly government-funded sector, work became increasingly hard to source and more sporadic. It was at this time that LDNM engaged a loyal following and the brand started to become established. It became increasingly difficult to balance legal work and the creation and growth of LDNM. At the same time that this trade-off was occurring, my father was diagnosed with lung cancer, and I soon found myself as a carer, lawyer and aspiring entrepreneur! I spent hours caring for my father, but with it being a digital company, I could be by his side and work on LDNM at the same time. It became a way to channel my emotions from what was happening. Dad took an active interest in the growing company; he was proud of us. A little over three months down the line, my father passed away following a truly savage battle with cancer. I was left holding a family together, but more determined than ever to make LDNM a success that he would be so proud of…

LDNM is now a way of life for me. I may have swapped professions, and a barrister's wig for an equally awful haircut, but the work ethic is the same: this is a full-time, night and day, working commitment that is growing and evolving on a daily basis.

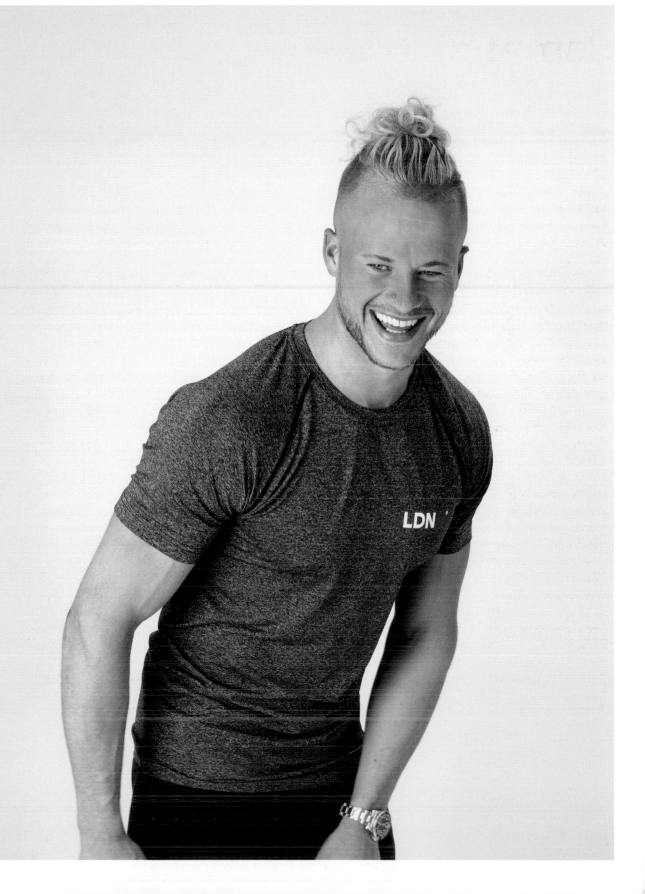

How to use this book

||||||||||||||||||||||||||||||||||||||||||||||||||||||||||||||||||||||||||||||||||||||||||||||

This book is broken up into four sections:
    Getting Started: setting your goals
    Leaner: diet and recipes
    Fitter: fitness
    Stronger: mindset and lifestyle

GETTING STARTED asks you to set your goals according to the SMART guide. Here, you will measure yourself, not just on the scales, but also by using the tape measure and progress selfies. You'll determine how much weight you want to lose, or muscle you want to gain, by calculating your BMR and TDEE, and we'll decode some diet and fitness jargon. We'll also tell you that success shouldn't be measured by a number, and that you can be successful at any size.

LEANER is where we will look at diet and the importance of macros, dispel some myths and set you up for success with some delicious kick-ass recipes that are healthy, nutritious and look great on your plate.

FITTER gives you the building blocks for weight-loss or muscle-gain success. You'll be introduced to HIIT (high-intensity interval training), which is great for improving your fitness and cardiovascular health, and to exercises that you can do outside, with a buddy, or in the gym. Plus we give you fitness routines for whatever level of fitness you're at.

STRONGER focuses on mindset and lifestyle. It acknowledges that becoming healthy and fit is an ongoing process that needs planning and perseverance to succeed. It looks at motivation, what it is, what kinds there are, and how to keep it going if you reach the dreaded plateau. It looks at changes to your lifestyle that you can make that don't mean giving up going out with your friends or eating the kinds of foods you love. It looks at incremental gains and how you can use them to get the results you want.

LET'S DO THIS THING!

Getting started

||||||||||||||||||||||||||||||||||||||||||||||||||||||||||||||||||||||||||

If you're anything like us, as soon as you decide that you want to get healthier, eat better, feel fitter and look great, you'll want to start right away. We understand that need to get started as quickly as possible.

First, however, you need to lay down the foundation for your new and improved active lifestyle. You need to set goals, SMART achievable goals that will give you something to aim for. You need to give yourself a baseline by which to measure your progress, and then you have to work out how much weight you want to lose or muscle you want to gain.

" The sooner
you start
the sooner
you'll see
the results "

MEASURING YOUR PROGRESS

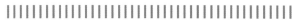

If we want to lose weight or gain muscle, the natural thing to do is jump on the scales. It's what we've been conditioned to do, after all, as many diet companies and weight-loss regimens see weight as the best indicator of progress.

But it's not a great indicator of progress. And it can be very dispiriting to be doing the work and feeling better in yourself, only to have the scales tell you otherwise. Weight fluctuates so much during the day and over time and can change due to so many factors – how hydrated you are, what clothes you wear, what time of the month it is if you're a woman… the list goes on and on.

Before you start, however, you need to take baseline measurements so that you can track your progress.

First of all, you should always track your weight and measurements at the same time of day every few days or week; if you need to, set a reminder on your phone. Wear the same clothes and make sure that your scales are on a flat and steady surface, ideally on the same spot each week, to get an accurate reading! Make sure you have a pen and paper handy to record your weight, or use an app on your phone (LDNM have a good one!), if that's more convenient for you.

Once you've weighed yourself, break out the measuring tape and measure the following: bust/chest (at widest point), waist measurement and hip measurement.

To find your waist measurement, locate the bottom of your ribs with your fingers and then find the tops of your hips. Make sure you're not holding your breath and take your waist measurement at the middle point. Write it down.

To find your hip measurement, stand in front of a mirror and put the measuring tape around your hips at the widest point. You might need to recruit a friend to help you with this.

You can write down your baseline measurements here:

Weight: _____
Bust/chest: _____
Waist: _____
Hip: _____

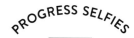

PROGRESS SELFIES

An important – and fun – way to measure your progress is through the progress selfie, which you can take after you weigh and measure yourself. You can take a few of these – front on, side on, from behind (if you can) – and compare them from week to week. Progress selfies will show you, beyond a doubt, that your hard work is paying off, even when the scales seem stuck!

WEIGHT LOSS

||||||||||||||||||||||||||||||||||||||||||||||||||||

When people talk about wanting to lose weight, what they usually mean is losing body fat. Losing fat isn't simply depriving yourself of food. There's so much more to it, especially if you want to continue to lose weight and do so in a healthy and enjoyable way, and then maintain it once you've hit your target. There is no quick fix when it comes to losing weight. Extreme measures aren't the answer, nor is simply guessing what you should eat or blindly following the latest fitness fad on social media. Here's a simplified but thorough approach to working out what you personally should be consuming.

Fat loss has a very simple rule, one that is common to every single weight-loss 'diet': that it places you in a caloric deficit. To lose weight, you consume fewer calories than your body is expending.

That's it. No rocket science. No superfoods, avocados or 'slimming' teas have the power to make you lose fat if you aren't in a calorie deficit (and they won't make you lose more fat even if you are!). You could just eat fast food and still lose body fat if you are in a calorie deficit, although we don't advise this as it isn't good for your health.

We are all unique. The number of calories one person consumes to lose weight can cause another to gain weight, due to different body size, body composition and amount of activity. Therefore the amount of calories you need to eat to lose weight will be individual to you.

To find the number of calories you need to consume to lose weight, we need to roughly calculate your maintenance calories – the number of calories you burn every day going about your usual business – and decrease from there.

The first step in doing this is to calculate your BMR (Basal Metabolic Rate) – the amount of calories your body needs to simply maintain normal bodily functions such as digestion, temperature regulation and respiration when you're at rest. Basically, the number of calories you would use if you were lying down in bed all day.

BODY FAT %

HOW TO FIND IT

You don't need to have an exact calculation here, as this is a very inexact science. The average body fat for men is between 15–20 per cent and is between 22–28 per cent for women. If you are below average body fat you should use a lower number, whereas if you are above average you should use a higher number.

As long as you are able to guesstimate your percentage you will be able to calculate your BMR reasonably accurately.

There are numerous different calculations but we prefer the Katch-McArdle formula:

BMR = 370 + (21.6 x lean mass in kilograms)

Once you have your BMR you need to multiply it by your 'activity factor', which takes into account the extra calories your body uses in your day-to-day life, including your exercise regime.

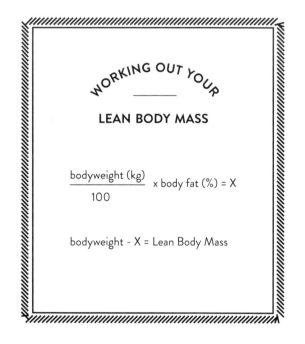

WORKING OUT YOUR
___

LEAN BODY MASS

$$\frac{\text{bodyweight (kg)}}{100} \times \text{body fat (\%)} = X$$

bodyweight - X = Lean Body Mass

FIND YOUR ACTIVITY FACTOR

SEDENTARY
BMR X 1.2
(sedentary work/daily routine, little or no additional exercise)

LIGHTLY ACTIVE
BMR X 1.3
(inactive work/daily routine and light exercise/sports 2–4 days per week)

MODERATELY ACTIVE
BMR X 1.5
(moderately active work/daily routine, exercise/sports 3–5 days per week)

VERY ACTIVE
BMR X 1.7
(active work/daily routine, hard exercise/ sports 6–7 days per week)

EXTREMELY ACTIVE
BMR X 1.9
(hard daily work/daily routine, exercise/ sports twice a day, full-time athlete, etc.)

If in doubt, choose a lower activity factor. For example, if you train twice daily but otherwise have an inactive routine, use an activity factor of 1.7.

This will now give you what is known as your TDEE – which is your **Total Daily Energy Expenditure** – this is the number of calories you require to maintain your body weight at your current activity level.

For example, Laura weighs 78 kilograms and has determined that she has an average percentage of body fat, which she works out as 25 per cent. Her job requires her to sit at her desk for most of the day, but she does take a short walk every lunchtime and goes to a Zumba class three times a week, giving her an activity factor of 'lightly active'. Let's do the maths.

First of all, Laura calculates her lean mass. This is her body weight in kilograms (78kg) divided by 100 (0.78) and then multiplied by her body fat percentage (25%), which gives her a total of 19.5. She then subtracts that number from her weight: 78 – 19.5 = 58.5. This means that her lean body mass is 58.5 kg.

With this number, she can now work out her BMR: 370 + (21.6 x 58.5) = 1,634 BMR.

This means that Laura needs to consume 1,634 calories per day just to maintain her body's normal functions.

Now let's find Laura's TDEE. As she is currently lightly active, we need to multiply her BMR of 1,634 by 1.3, giving her a total of 2,124 calories, which is the number of calories she needs to consume in a day to maintain her weight given her current rate of activity.

To lose fat you need to eat less than your TDEE to place you in a caloric deficit. But just how much?

HOW MUCH OF A DEFICIT SHOULD YOU BE IN TO ACHIEVE FAT LOSS?

||||||||||||||||||||||||||||||||||||||||||||||||||

20% BELOW MAINTENANCE
conservative deficit (good starting point for people who have average body-fat level)

25% BELOW MAINTENANCE
moderate deficit (good starting point for those with above-average body-fat levels)

30% BELOW MAINTENANCE
aggressive deficit (maximum fat loss – recommended for obese and time-sensitive deadlines, although possible weight regain afterwards if diet is not controlled)

Let's look at Laura again. She has determined that she has average body fat and is happy to lose weight at a slower and more sustainable pace. She decides that she is going to consume 20 per cent fewer calories per day. Twenty per cent of her TDEE of 2,214 is 425. Subtracting 425 from 2,124 gives her 1,699. Let's be generous and give her an extra calorie, making the total number of calories she needs for a conservative rate of weight loss as 1,700 calories per day.

WHAT IS A REALISTIC RATE OF WEIGHT LOSS?

||||||||||||||||||||||||||||||||||||||||||||

0.5–1.5% OF TOTAL BODY WEIGHT PER WEEK.

We have found this is a realistic level to aim for. The more body fat you have and the newer you are to training, the more body fat you can lose, which means – at the start of your programme at least – the nearer you are likely to be to the 1.5%.

As your body-fat levels decrease and you become more conditioned to training, the amount of body fat you lose each week will begin to drop.

Laura, for example, is 78 kilograms, which is equivalent to 172 pounds. In her first week, she can expect to lose between 0.39 and 1.13kg. As she loses weight, that range will decrease.

Remember that your weight isn't the only measure of your body's changing shape. If it seems that you're not losing weight quickly, check out your measurements and take a look at your progress selfies and see how they change over time.

MUSCLE BUILDING

||||||||||||||||||||||||||||||||||||||||||||

If losing weight requires a calorie deficit, building muscle requires the opposite – a calorie surplus – that's to say you consume more calories than you expend. We will look at this topic in simple detail here, our guides however explore other key variables such as body type and macro splits, and meal timings.

Once again, to build muscle you need to work out your BMR, then TDEE, before you can be sure to place yourself into a surplus (see pages 24–25).

Once you have your TDEE, you simply need add the amounts below:

MEN
initially add 250 calories as your surplus and then 50kcal every 2 weeks.

WOMEN
initially add 125 calories as your surplus and then 30kcal every 2 weeks.

WHAT IS A REALISTIC RATE OF MUSCLE GAIN?

||||||||||||||||||||||||||||||||||||||||||||

It depends on your starting point. A slower rate is likely for those already accustomed to training, and a quicker rate for those new to training.

BEGINNER
1–1.5% of body weight per month.

INTERMEDIATE
0.5–1% of body weight per month.

ADVANCED
0.25–0.5% of body weight per month.

With these numbers in mind it's easy to set realistic expectations and goals

SET YOUR GOAL

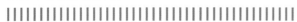

Each journey ends with a destination, and when you start out on your fitness programme, you need to have a clear and specific goal in mind. It's not enough to simply want to lose weight or build muscle, you need to decide exactly what you want to achieve and set a time frame. It's helpful to set your goal according to the SMART method.

SMART GOALS

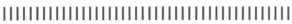

To help make your goal as clear as possible, use the SMART method. SMART stands for the following:

S   specific
M   measureable
A   action-orientated
R   realistic
T   time-based

Thinking of your goal in this way makes it much more 'real', and easier to 'visualise' (see page 264). It makes sure that you're not dooming yourself to fail by choosing goals that are unrealistic. And it sets a time-frame, so that you can see that there's an end in sight.

Let's say you're a woman who is five foot eight and weighs 78 kilograms. Your goal might be the following:

S   to lose 10 kilograms
M   by measuring my bust, waist and hip measurements, taking a progress selfie, and jumping on the scales
A   doing the beginner's HIIT programme 2x a week, doing the beginner's strength training 3x a week, making sure I eat a satisfying breakfast every day, tracking my food and training every day
R   10 kilograms is in the middle of the BMI charts for a healthy weight
T   I would like to lose five kilos by my best friend's wedding in three months' time

YOUR GOAL

Now that you've decided on a goal according to the SMART method, here's a space to write it down. At the back of this book we've also included a SMART template for you to photocopy and stick somewhere you see every day – perhaps on a mirror or the door of your fridge.

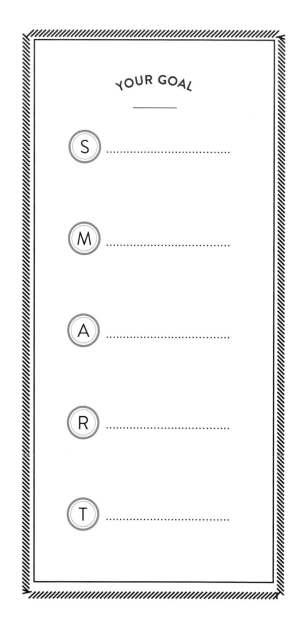

YOUR GOAL

S ....

M ....

A ....

R ....

T ....

KEYWORDS, ACRONYMS AND BUZZWORDS DECODED

DIETARY

CLEAN EATING
Only eating so-called 'clean' foods as an approach to weight loss. For the record, 'clean' is not a word we use to describe foods or how we eat; demonising or glorifying foods and entire food groups is not only unfounded, it can cause damaging negative associations around eating. Foods in themselves don't make you fat or thin, total calories does.

CHEAT MEAL
A meal that is outside of your intended calorie allowance, either intentionally or unintentionally.

FLEXIBLE DIETING
A method allowing you to integrate any food type of your preference into your total calorie intake allowance, while not disregarding the need for a healthy approach to your diet.

IIFYM
The antithesis of clean eating: eating anything you want, so long as it hits your macros.

MACROS
Abbreviation of 'macronutrients' – the major nutrients that provide energy/calories. The three main macros are protein, carbohydrates and fat.

TRAINING

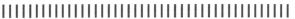

BULKING
A widely used term to describe the process of increasing calorie intake, to place you in a calorie surplus, the goal being primarily to build muscle.

CUTTING
Another widely used term to describe the process of reducing calories, to place you in a calorie deficit, the goal being to shed body fat, and create a lean body.

DOMS
Or 'delayed onset muscle soreness' is the pain you often experience the day(s) after a session.

FAILURE
When you physically can't perform an exercise any more.

FORM/TECHNIQUE
The prescribed way/best practice to do an exercise to mitigate the chance of an injury.

GAINS
A term used to describe the increase in muscle mass or weight.

HIIT
High-intensity interval training. An interval-based training protocol said to have an after-burn effect for up to 48 hours after exercise.

REPETITION
One completed movement.

SETS
The amount of continuous reps you do is called a set.

TEMPO
The speed at which you lift during the exercise.

OTHER

STRONG NOT SKINNY
Placing an emphasis on getting fit, healthy and strong, rather than extreme low-calorie diets that focus merely on an idealised weight. Skinny doesn't necessarily equal healthy.

SUCCESS AT ANY SIZE
||||||||||||||||||||||||||||||||||||||||

'Success at any size' is a mantra you'll see throughout this book. It means exactly what it says: you don't need to reach a certain size or attain a certain physique to be successful. Society has a very narrow perceived view of what is desirable or beautiful for men and women, a view so narrow it's unobtainable for most of us. Given the number of photoshopping stories that are around, it's even unobtainable for the models and actors held up as society's ideals!

We're two sets of brothers – including one set of twins – and none of us has exactly the same body type, and none of us wants to look exactly the same as the others. We've all taken different paths on the road to fitness, and we all have encountered different challenges along the way. We're not cookie-cutter personalities, we don't have cookie-cutter bodies, and we don't expect our followers to look exactly the same or to want the exact-same things as each other.

People come in all shapes and sizes, and the number on the scales doesn't say anything about you as a person. All it says is what you weigh; nothing more, nothing less. It says nothing about your sense of humour or your intelligence or your personality. So don't be a slave to it. Use the scales as a tool but remember their limitations – weight can fluctuate from day to day, even from hour to

hour – don't weigh yourself too often, and don't get hung up on the number. Find other indicators to show that you're progressing – your clothes are looser, your measurements are smaller, you can do that set of repetitions more easily than you could a week ago and you're ready to move up to the next level of training. These are much better ways to show how you're progressing along your fitness journey.

Your body is the ultimate multi-tasker. As you're reading this, it's performing a huge number of conscious and unconscious actions, from breathing to blinking to digesting your breakfast, to telling you when you're hungry or thirsty. And all this while you're taking in information through your eyes and interpreting it in your brain. Sure, you want to feel better in your clothes, you want to be healthy, you want to feel leaner, fitter, stronger, and that's all good. Just don't let anyone tell you that your body is less than amazing.

All we want from you is for you to be happy in your own skin. To be positive about what you have accomplished in your quest for a healthy body. To see obstacles as challenges, and to persevere with your plan if you have the odd setback. We want you to enjoy doing the things you love to do for as long as possible. We want you to be healthy and we want you to have fun.

Let's do it. Let's get Leaner, Fitter, Stronger.

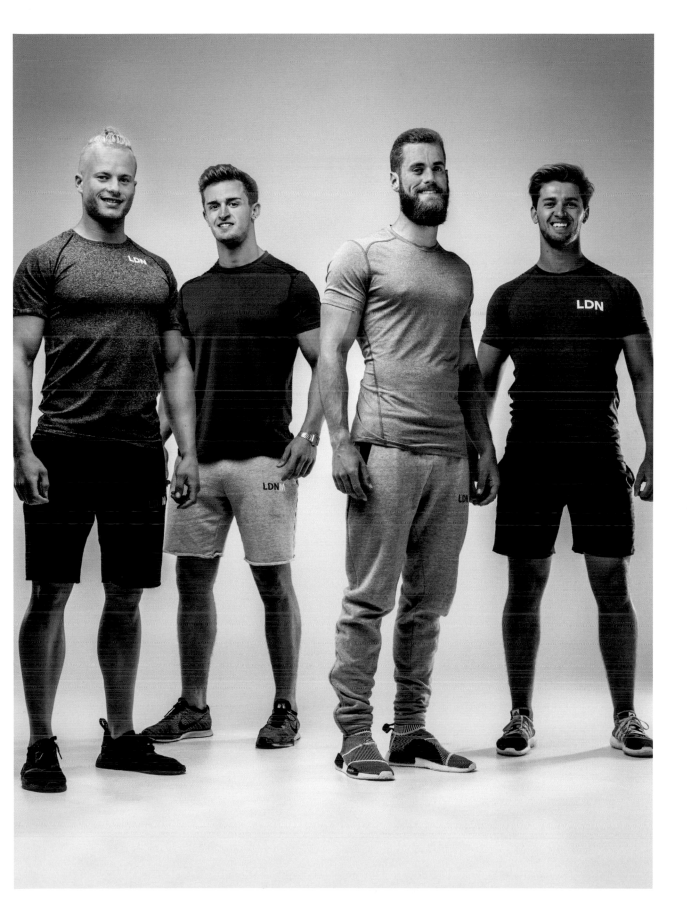

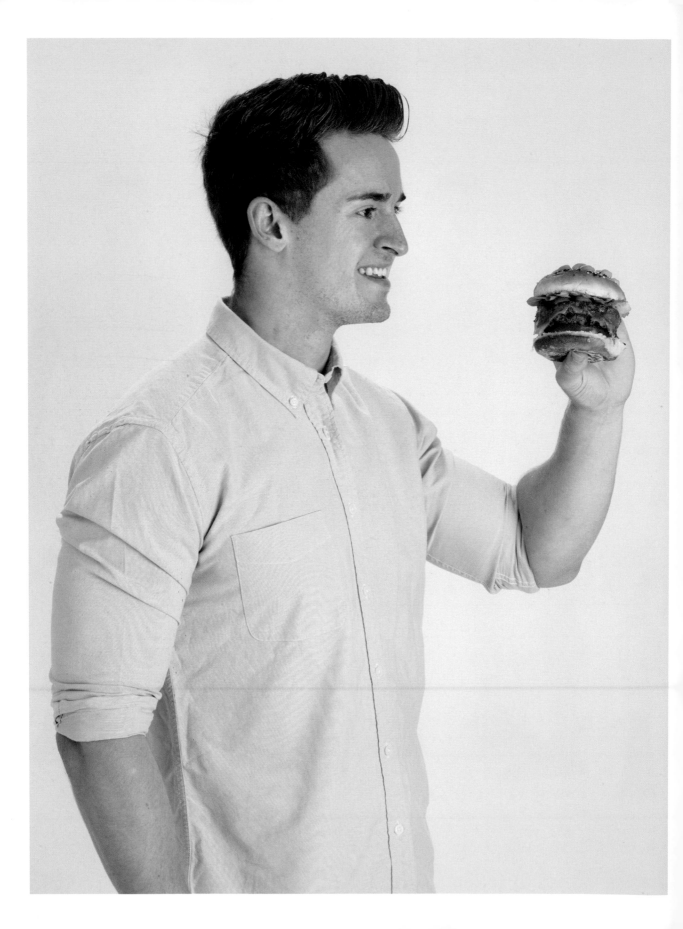

LEANER

||||||||||||||||||||||||||||||||||||||||||||||||||||||||||||||||||||||

You've chosen this book because you want to change. You've set your weight-loss or muscle-gaining goals (see page 28) and you're all fired up and ready to go. And here is where you should start, with your diet, the foods you put in to fuel your body.

Diet is crucial. In fact, it's the most important part of any training programme. You could do any number of planks, sit-ups or cardio sessions, but the plain truth of the matter is that without a good diet plan in place, you will not achieve the results that you want.

When we say 'diet', we don't mean banning certain food groups. We don't believe in 'good' foods and 'bad' foods. We certainly don't believe that you should refuse that glass of wine at your office party. No, By 'diet' we mean the food that you put into your body. If you want to change your body and make that change permanent, you need to change your lifestyle, and your diet is a large part of that.

To become leaner, fitter, stronger, you will probably have to reset the way you think about food. You may think of food in terms of 'reward' and 'punishment'. You reward yourself for getting through a hard day with a chocolate bar; you punish yourself for overeating with a green salad. Or you might think of food as 'comfort', something that you turn to when you're feeling sad or lonely or bored. You may be a foodie and are worried that a change in diet will mean that you'll have to give up the foods that you love.

Food is fuel, it's as simple as that. If you use food as a reward, find something else that you can use to treat yourself with. If you've thrown your diet plan out of the window one day, simply go back to eating well the next – don't try to limit your food intake in an effort to make up for a day off the plan. If you're eating food for comfort, identify what it is that's bothering or worrying you and address that. If you're a foodie, well, we've got good news. The food in our recipe section is delicious, nutritious and looks great on your plate. Yes, food is primarily fuel for your body, but there's no reason why it can't be tasty and enjoyable to eat too!

TRACK YOUR WEEK

||||||||||||||||||||||||||||||||||||||||||||||

How well do you know what you eat? Do you make conscious choices or do you just grab what you can, when you can? Chances are, if you want to lose weight, you've probably not thought much about what you've eaten during the day. It's amazing how much and what you can consume when you're not thinking about it.

You're likely to be raring to go with the diet plan, but before then it's a good idea to track what you eat and when, over seven days. You can either use a food-tracking app on your phone, or go analogue with a piece of paper, or photocopy the tracker at the end of this book. Don't judge yourself during this week, and don't cheat – this is a very useful tool for working out when you eat well and where you can improve. It can also show you flashpoints throughout the day. Do you start off the day with a good breakfast? Do you have breakfast at all? Do you have a chocolate bar at 3pm because you're feeling tired and need something to perk you up? What happens at the end of the day – do you cook food from scratch, or do you only have time and energy for a ready-meal?

Finding out what your pattern of eating is will help you work out how you can fit your new diet in around your lifestyle. During the week, you might need ideas for breakfasts you can make while you rush out the door; if you come home from work late, what meals can you prepare in advance or whip up in a few minutes to avoid relying on ready-meals or takeaways?

At the end of the week, take a look at your tracker and see if any patterns emerge. Do you eat well from Monday to Friday but you find weekends are when you overindulge? Do you go out after work for 'just one' with your colleagues, and it ends up becoming a bit of a session? If you can work out what your flashpoints are, then you can find strategies to put in place to avoid them.

You will need to think about the food you put into your body a lot at the start of your Leaner, Fitter, Stronger journey, but soon you will find that you will automatically make better choices.

'GOOD' VS 'BAD' FOODS

The weight-loss industry in the UK is worth around £2 billion a year. This means that as a society, we spend an awful lot of money on something that rarely works. Most weight-loss companies rely on repeat business to make money, which means that people who have lost weight return to the plan that failed them once the kilos start piling on again. This leads to yo-yo dieting and, more often than not, you end up weighing much more than when you started the diet.

Weight-loss products tend to focus on restricting one type of food group or another, promoting the idea that one type of food is better or worse than another. And that thinking can be pretty hard to shake. For years, fat was the enemy. Then it was carbs. But fat and carbohydrates play an important part in a balanced diet. What's most important is the percentage of protein, fat and carbohydrates that you put in your body.

Try to release yourself from the mindset that one food is better or worse than another. If you really enjoy chocolate, pop the occasional bar into your eating plan. If you want to go out for dinner with your friends, factor that in to your weekly food planner.

We mentioned so-called 'clean' eating on page 28 and will talk about it again on page 40 – this is because everywhere we look it seems like something else is branded a 'clean juice' or a 'dirty burger'; yes clean *rhymes* with lean, but it does not equal lean. The myth of clean is misleading about what constitutes healthy eating and can be harmful; approach with caution.

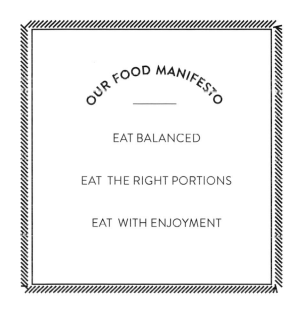

OUR FOOD MANIFESTO

EAT BALANCED

EAT THE RIGHT PORTIONS

EAT WITH ENJOYMENT

SUPPLEMENTS

We see supplements as just that, a supplement to your diet and nutrition to allow you to either increase your intake of a certain element, or to increase the convenience of doing so.

Many sports nutrition companies have unrealistic claims for their products that are easy to buy in to and which don't deliver (we know – before we knew better, we bought into these claims ourselves!). If you see a claim for a product that seems too good to be true, it usually is.

If you think of your diet as a pyramid, what should be at the very bottom is a balanced diet including all the macros. What's next is sports nutrition, and then at the very top are supplements. These should be used to back up your healthy-eating plan, not used as a substitute for it.

We've engineered our own LDNM supplements for this very reason. Our supplements are of the highest quality at an affordable price. Unlike other companies we don't stock thousands of miracle-promising products. Rather, we only sell a core range of products that have proven effects when used as part of a good diet and training plan and offer a tangible benefit for our users.

These are the core supplements that we use, rate and recommend and which form part of our LDNM supplement range (https://supps.ldnmuscle.com).

Whey protein

Whey is high-quality protein derived from cow's milk. When milk turns and separates into curds and liquid, whey protein is suspended in the liquid and isolated by an industrial process.

Whey doesn't have magic power to build muscle as some companies claim; we prefer to think of it as a food rather than a supplement. It's a great convenience tool to help increase and reach your desired protein intake at a meal, or as part of a meal replacement when you are on the go. A fair few of the recipes in this book use whey as an ingredient and we do recommend you go with our LDNM products; yes we are biaised, but if we trust it, you can too.

Some companies sell 'whey blends', which often means they are using cheaper proteins to bulk out their powders, so always check the ingredients list and avoid products laced with inferior proteins such as soy and wheat.

If you are lactose intolerant or vegan, a good-quality hemp or pea protein (ideally a 'vegan blend') is the best alternative to whey.

Instant oats

Instant oats are another supplement we suggest as a great convenience food to help reach your desired carbohydrate intake at a meal, to add extra carbohydrates or as part of a meal replacement when on the go.

As they are dense in carbohydrates, you only have to consume a small amount to take in a high amount of carbohydrates.

If you find the taste horrible, mix them with a little Nesquik, flavoured protein powder or flavouring drops.

Creatine (Creapure)

Creatine monohydrate is the most-studied supplement in sport science and is 100 per cent effective and safe. It saturates your muscles' stores of creatine phosphate, which allows them to retain more energy for explosive, anaerobic activities such as lifting, jumping and sprinting.

Creapure is a high-purity creatine monohydrate; no other creatine supplement will be more effective, regardless of price or marketing. Supplementing with 3–5g mixed in water with your post-workout meal or breakfast will achieve 100 per cent saturation of your muscles. There is no need for a 'loading phase', which may lead to bloating and gastrointestinal discomfort for some people.

Caffeine

You can get caffeine from tea, coffee, energy drinks or caffeine tablets/powder.

If supplementing with tablets/powder, start with 100mg of caffeine before a session and steadily increase your dose each session until you find your optimal intake. Don't take more than 400mg a day in total.

Caffeine powder tastes terrible, so we advise mixing it with squash to mask the taste!

Pre-workout

Sometimes attracting bad press, pre-workouts have had their fair share of media scares. For those with a high caffeine tolerance, or when you are in dire need of an energy boost, these drinks can power you through the workout you didn't want to do. We see our pre-workout more as a rescue remedy than something you should become reliant on.

BCAAs

BCAAs, or branched chain amino acids, is a protein supplement. We prefer powdered BCAAs to pill form.

Supplement with 5–10g of BCAA powder during your workout. We advise adding squash to improve the taste if the powder is unflavoured!

You only need to take BCAAs during your workout. Supplementing with them outside of your workout will have little or no effect as you should already be eating enough protein to maximise protein synthesis.

Multivitamin

Multivitamins cannot replace nutrients and vitamins from whole foods.

They are good to ensure you are consuming the necessary amount of vitamins and minerals such as potassium and vitamin B12, which are deficient in many people's diets.

Long-term studies as to the benefits of multivitamins are currently inconclusive, but they are not harmful and are inexpensive so are worth supplementing your daily diet.

Vitamin D3

The majority of the population is deficient in vitamin D, which can lead to a decrease in bone density and an increased risk of cardiovascular disease and several different cancers.

Supplementing with 1000–4000IU of vitamin D per day is widely considered safe and effective.

Supplement vitamin D at breakfast or any meal throughout the day.

Omega-3

Omega-3 is a fatty acid that's normally found in oily fish, seeds and full-fat dairy products.

These fatty acids are said to be essential to the normal functioning of the heart and brain and may also aid joint health and even help promote fat loss.

" Be realistic, remain motivated "

FLEXIBLE DIETING

We feel very strongly that a diet that restricts the food that you enjoy isn't going to be sustainable in the long term. If you love ice cream, for example, there's no point in denying yourself the occasional cone if you're going to feel deprived without it. If you want ice cream, factor it into your diet plan and enjoy! You'll be more likely to stick to your plan if you're not craving 'forbidden' foods.

Flexible dieting means that you can eat whatever foods you like within your plan, so long as you stick to your assigned calories most of the time. If you have calories to use up at the end of the day, weigh out that ice cream so that it matches the calories you have left and enjoy!

If you're going out to eat, check the website of the restaurant you're eating at – many these days include the calorie and nutrition content on their menus. This makes it easy to factor in a meal out with your normal diet. You might want to lower your calories and carbohydrates for a couple of meals beforehand too, if that puts your mind at rest.

Don't think of your new eating plan as 'Life vs Diet', think of it as a healthy, sustainable and enjoyable part of your new lifestyle.

MYTH BUSTING

Weight loss is the best indicator of progress
While you should monitor your weight at regular intervals, it shouldn't be the only type of measurement you use, and you shouldn't get too hung up on the numbers. What's much more helpful – and more fun to see as your body becomes healthier – is taking progress selfies and body measurements. Progress selfies will show you beyond a doubt that your body is changing, even if the numbers on the scales are not moving downwards as fast as you'd like.

So many things can affect your weight – how hydrated you are, how much food you've eaten, what time of day or month it is, even the weather! So take your three measurements at the same time every week or fortnight. Choose what day is best for you and pop a reminder in your calendar. Try to make the conditions that you weigh yourself in as similar as possible – wear the same clothes, choose whether to measure yourself before or after a meal – and stick to it.

Carbohydrates cause you to gain fat
Carbohydrate consumption alone does not cause you to gain fat. You do not need to cut out carbs in order to lose weight, and cutting out carbs altogether will lead to poor-quality training and mental performance. You are also more likely to binge on foods you have cut out, and this can also make you more prone to mood swings.

You gain fat by one simple rule: on a regular basis you eat more calories per day than you need to maintain your weight. These excess calories are stored as body fat.

Remember that calories are a measure of energy, so if you expend more calories than you consume – i.e., on a regular basis you eat fewer calories than you need to maintain your weight – you will lose weight.

You need to cut out bad foods

When considering only fat or weight loss and gain, food type is not imperative – total calories are. This means you do not need to cut out 'bad foods' entirely.

Including traditionally 'bad foods' within a calorie-controlled diet that is balanced and varied will not have negative health effects, and will increase the likelihood of you sticking to your diet plan. This consistency will allow you to improve your body composition without degrading your quality of life.

We feel reducing body fat and enjoying a flexible diet to be healthier than yo-yoing in weight due to clean diets and periods of no diet due to hating your previous clean diet and needing a break!

You must cook every meal

Again this is complete nonsense. You can absolutely opt for shop-bought sandwiches, express rices and even ready-meals from time to time. Including these within a balanced diet is totally fine. We aren't advocating a diet based on processed foods, but don't beat yourself up if here and there you take a cooking short-cut.

Lots of people simply do not have time to search the supermarkets for niche, expensive ingredients or spend hours cooking. Do not feel you have to cook a masterpiece each time. In our recipe section you'll find a number of tasty and nutritious meal ideas that won't take up all of your time!

You must 'eat clean' to lose fat

'Eating clean' has become a buzzword in the health and training community. But what is 'eating clean'? It means different things to different people, but it's widely understood by the general public to mean a diet consisting of only traditionally healthy foods. What makes a diet healthy, though, is very subjective. Does it include grains? Meat? Dairy products? What about sugar? What about fat? Often 'eating clean' is endorsed by a celebrity or food writer, and they're often very restrictive.

We think that cutting out foods that you enjoy because you think they're not part of an 'eating clean' regimen is ultimately destined to fail. You don't need to exist on plain chicken and steamed veggies in order to achieve your fitness and aesthetic goals. You can include the foods that you enjoy within your diet, as long as your diet is balanced and calorie controlled. Remember what we said above: burning more calories than you take in will make you lose weight.

You can't put on fat on a 'clean diet'

Some fitness bloggers and celebrities will say they lost weight because they 'cleaned up their diet', but in reality they will have cut calories by banning a list of foods (that they probably enjoy). This also gives the wrong message that you cannot gain body fat on a clean diet.

Again it's simple: if you eat too many calories per day from chicken, avocado and rye bread you will gain fat. On the other hand, if you know your calorie target for the day, choose to eat spaghetti bolognese and sandwiches but keep within your target, you will lose weight.

You shouldn't eat carbs after 6pm

This is rubbish, especially if you are training later in the day (or have trouble sleeping). As we mentioned previously, fat or weight gain and loss are dependent on total calories for the day – regardless of whether these come from carbs, fats and protein, or fats and protein alone.

If you are training in the evening you will likely have carbs in the evening, before and after your workout, for fuel and for replenishment. This is the smart thing to do, and carbs will not simply turn to fat after a certain hour of the day. Carbohydrates in your last meal of the day have also been shown to aid sleep due to the hormones they cause your body to release.

Protein powder is only for bodybuilders

Protein powder will not make you bulky, and is not solely for male bodybuilders. Whey protein shakes and suchlike are a handy convenience tool when a meal isn't an option, or when the protein-based part of a meal isn't sufficient.

Protein powders can be consumed at any point during the day, and are not only for pre- or post-workout, and certainly not for during your training as some companies or individuals suggest.

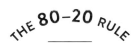

THE 80–20 RULE

Very simply put, the 80–20 rule means that if you eat healthy, nutritious food 80 per cent of the time you can eat foods you would typically consider 'off limits' in a diet for the other 20 per cent.

Be careful though – spread that 20 per cent over a week, rather than having a binge on one day. We don't advise having 'cheat days' because 'cheating' with your food is an example of the 'good food, bad food' dichotomy we want you to avoid. Plan that 20 per cent just as you would the 80 per cent. That way, you can enjoy everything you eat without guilt.

Skinny teas work

Skinny teas and fat burners are both ineffective and not worth the money, in our opinion. Detox, skinny and gym teas are simply green teas spiced up with some exotic ingredients and some even have a mild laxative effect.

Note how they only provide the 'desired effect' when combined with the suggested diet and training advice, which consists of minimal calories and lots of exercise. Combine this with a diuretic and mild laxative and it isn't surprising that people achieve weight loss and attribute it to the tea alone! This is when in reality they would have experienced the same results without the tea, just by training frequently and eating a little less.

Quick fixes: detoxes, 7-day slims, crash diets

Quick fixes may work in the very short term, but when you revert to normal eating and training habits, more often than not you'll be in a worse position than you were at the beginning.

These fads – detoxes, 7-day slims, juice diets, etc. – put you in an unsustainable routine, and too large a caloric deficit. To put it simply, you progress in a manner you cannot maintain beyond a few weeks and once you revert to your normal habit you put the weight back on – and more!

Eating every 2–3 hours 'stokes the metabolic fire'

The original idea behind this was that eating little and often would keep your metabolism 'ticking over' so that you burn more calories from digesting food.

It turns out that your body burns the same amount of calories whether you eat X calories over one meal or seven meals, so meal frequency has no effect on body composition if total calories are controlled.

People who have fewer meals (two or less) may find themselves binge-eating and overconsuming calories more regularly due to the restriction of food and the build-up of hunger and food cravings.

We suggest three to five meals a day, depending on your preference and daily routine.

Cheat-day theories

The notion behind 'cheat days' is that you severely restrict your calorie intake for six days of the week and on the seventh eat whatever you like, without consequence, because it will 'spike your metabolism': you will burn more of the calories that you eat and also prevent adaptation of your metabolism to the reduced intake.

It has been shown that large spikes in calorie intake (a cheat day) during a period of dieting will have no lasting effect of increasing metabolism or preventing its adaption to the lower calorie intake.

Small daily increases in calories – also known as 'refeeds' can be useful during extended periods of dieting to ease the mental fatigue of calorie restriction and increase energy levels for particularly intense training days.

STOCKING UP

||||||||||||||||||||||||||||||||||||||||||

Here are a few things that we all like to keep in good supply in our kitchens; they form the bedrock of many of our meals and are great to have to hand for when time is short and inspiration limited!

STORE CUPBOARD

- Rolled oats – make a quick flour by blitzing in a food processor
- Tinned pulses – chickpeas, cannellini beans, kidney beans... endless possibilities!
- Olive oil
- Vinegar – we like balsamic and cider ones
- Coconut oil – don't feel you need to cook everything with this, as it can get very expensive, but it is great for baking
- Tinned tomatoes
- Nuts
- Nut-butter
- Brown rice
- Basmati rice
- Honey
- Maple syrup
- Soy sauce
- Sesame oil
- Rice wine vinegar
- Ground spices – the easiest way to add flavour to a dish; have a healthy supply of paprika, chilli, cumin, coriander, curry powder, oregano, basil, cinnamon and ginger and you'll never be far from a tasty meal
- Cornflour
- Tinned fish

FRIDGE

- Milk – cow's milk, nut milk, drinking coconut milk
- Butter
- Free-range eggs
- Hummus
- Cheese – feta, halloumi, mozzarella
- Chicken

FREEZER

- Loads of veggies – spinach, peas, edamame beans, mixed bags
- Fruit – the supermarket bags of berries are great for smoothies, and if you have any apples or bananas that are going a little off in the fruit bowl, chop them up and freeze them in some tupperware (peel the bananas first)
- Wholegrain bread
- Pitta bread
- Wholemeal wraps
- Frozen prawns, fish and a pack or two of mince (beef, turkey or Quorn)

Breakfast

||||||||||||||||||||||||||||||||||||||||||||||||||

Mexican food always hits the spot in our books, and this is our take on a classic recipe. It's quick and easy and makes a great (and much fresher) alternative to a fry-up. Equally good for a hangover too...

Huevos rancheros

||||||||||||||||||||||||||||||||||||||||||||||||||||||||||||||||||||||||||||||||||||||||||||||||||

// SERVES 2 //

2 tsp olive oil,
　plus extra for brushing
1 small onion, finely chopped
1 garlic clove, finely chopped
½ jalapeño, sliced or pinch
　of dried chilli flakes
1 red pepper, thinly sliced
400g tinned chopped tomatoes
1 tbsp tomato purée
½ tsp coconut sugar
2 wholemeal tortillas
2 eggs
coriander, chopped
sea salt and freshly ground black
　pepper

TO SERVE

1 avocado, destoned and diced
cherry tomatoes
grated Cheddar cheese
lime wedges

1 / Preheat the oven to 140°C/Gas 1.

2 / Heat the oil in a small cast-iron pan, add the onion and a pinch of salt. Cook over medium-low heat for 10 minutes, until softened but not browned. Add the garlic, jalapeño and red pepper and cook for another 5 minutes, just to soften the pepper a little.

3 / Add the tomatoes and tomato purée to the pan and stir together well. Add 50ml water and the sugar, bring to the boil and reduce the heat to very low. Let the tomatoes bubble away gently for 15–20 minutes, until reduced slightly and thickened. Season to taste with salt and pepper.

4 / Meanwhile, cut the tortillas into triangles or shards and brush with a little oil, and sprinkle with sea salt. Arrange on a baking tray, in a single layer, and bake for 3–6 minutes, or until brown and crisp. Turn them over once if needed.

5 / Once the sauce has thickened, use a wooden spoon to make two indentations in the sauce. Break the eggs into the holes. Simmer the eggs gently in the sauce, covered, for 8–10 minutes, or until the whites are opaque and the yolks still runny. Sprinkle with coriander.

6 / Serve in the pan with the tortilla chips, avocado, tomatoes, cheese and lime wedges on the side.

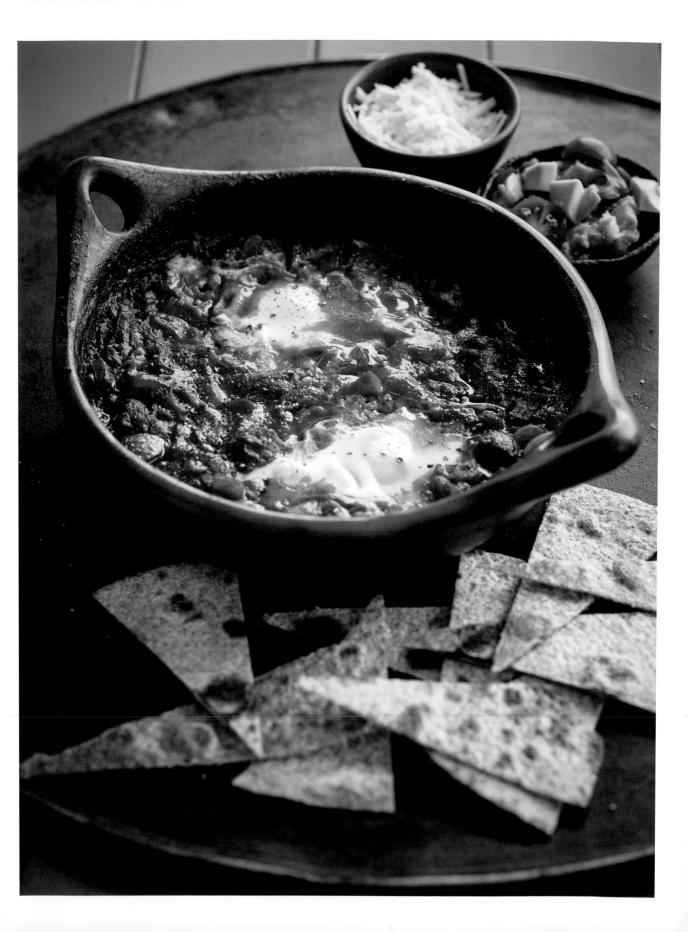

This makes a really good brunch dish for a lazy weekend when you have a little more time on your hands. Great with some French bread or muffins too to soak up all the tomatoey-cheesy-olive oil goodness.

Baked tomato with kale & goat's cheese

||||||||||||||||||||||||||||||||||||||||||||||||||||||||||||||||||||||||||||||||||||||||||||

// SERVES 3 //

6 firm, large vine tomatoes
large handful kale leaves,
    tough stalks discarded
1 garlic clove, crushed
1 egg
330g goat's cheese,
    roughly chopped
few chives, snipped
2 sprigs thyme, leaves picked
extra virgin olive oil
sea salt and freshly ground
    black pepper

1 / Preheat the oven to 180°C/Gas 4.

2 / Prepare the tomatoes by slicing the stem end off and reserving. Use a spoon to scoop out the seeds and tomato flesh, leaving just the shells. Put the tomatoes upside down on a paper towel to help drain out excess liquid.

3 / Roughly shred the kale leaves and put in a bowl with 2 tablespoons water. Cover and microwave for 2–3 minutes and leave to steam. The leaves should just be wilted. Drain the kale and put back in the bowl with the garlic, egg, goat's cheese, chives and thyme leaves. Mix together well.

4 / Place the tomatoes on a roasting tray. Sprinkle the insides of the tomatoes with salt and pepper and drizzle in a little olive oil. Spoon the goat's cheese mixture between the tomatoes, filling almost to the top. Pop the lids of the tomatoes on top and bake for 25–30 minutes, until the tomatoes are tender, slightly browned and the cheese oozing.

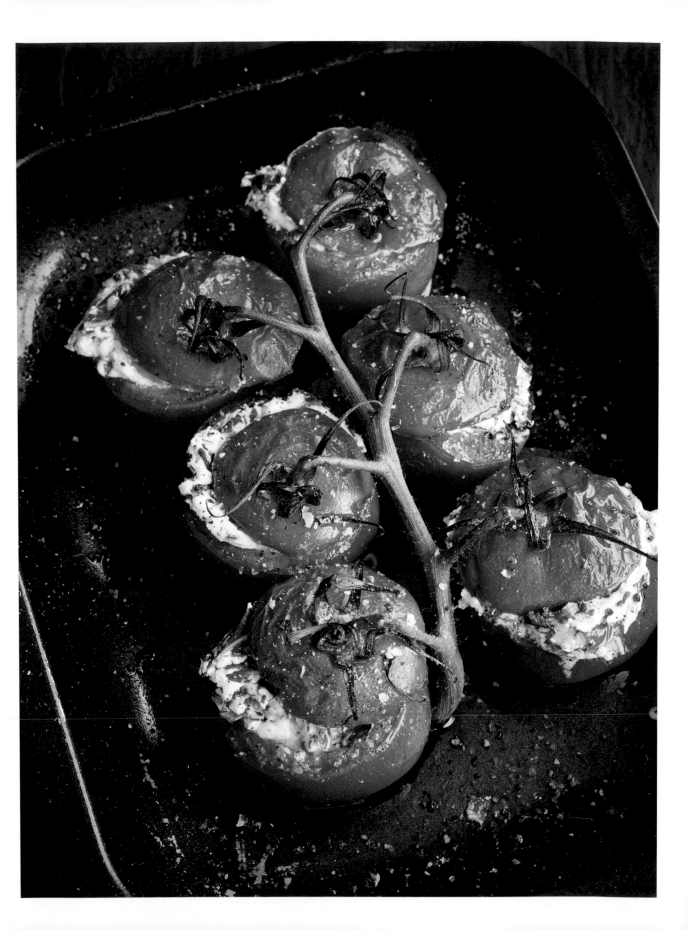

We love a smoothie at the LDNM headquarters; here are our four favourites. These recipes make a healthy-sized serving for one person.

Smoothies

||||||||||||||||||||||||||||||||||||||||||||||||||||||||||||||||||||||||||||||||||||||||||||||||||||||||||||||||||||||

ENERGY BOOSTER

1 frozen banana, peeled and sliced / 200ml nut milk or milk of choice / 1 scoop vanilla whey protein powder/ 1 tbsp peanut butter or cashew butter / 2 pinches ground cinnamon

Blitz in a blender and sprinkle with cinnamon to serve.

BERRY BOMB

large handful frozen mixed berries / 1 small banana, peeled and sliced / 200ml nut milk or coconut water / 1 tbsp almond or cashew butter / 1 tsp vanilla extract / 1 tsp agave syrup or honey / squeeze lime juice

Blitz the ingredients in a blender and serve.

THE GREEN ONE

1 ripe avocado / 1 small frozen banana, peeled and sliced / large handful frozen pineapple pieces / 3 large spinach leaves, roughly chopped / 1 kiwi fruit, peeled and roughly chopped/ 1 scoop vanilla LDNM whey protein powder/ 200ml almond milk (or milk of choice)

Slice the avocado in half, remove the stone and scoop the flesh into a blender or food processor. Add the banana, pineapple, spinach, kiwi, vanilla whey and milk. Blitz until smooth and drink immediately.

GINGERBREAD PROTEIN SHAKE

1 banana, peeled and sliced / pinch ground cinnamon / pinch ground cloves / ½ tsp ground ginger / 1 scoop vanilla LDNM whey protein powder / 250ml almond milk (or milk of choice) / handful ice cubes

Blitz the ingredients in a blender or food processor and drink immediately.

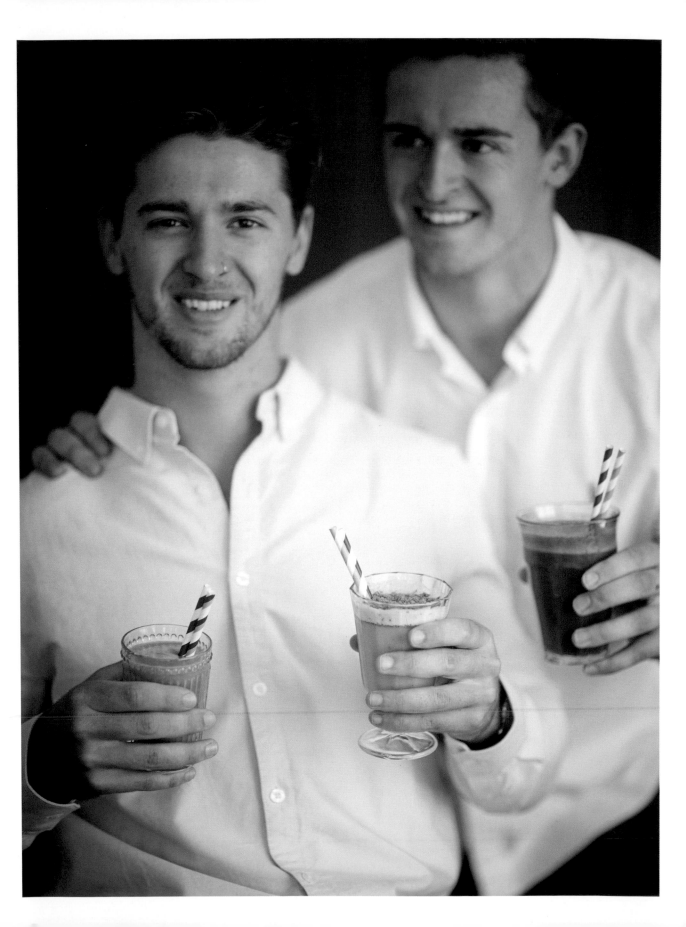

Our twist on a classic snack. Although normally associated with pubs and picnics, these make a great protein-packed and portable breakfast; they can be kept in the fridge for up to three days so make a batch on Sunday and you'll be laughing till hump-day.

Curried chicken Scotch eggs

||||||||||||||||||||||||||||||||||||||||||||||||||||||||||||||||||||||||||||||||||||||||||||||||||||||||||||||||||||||||||||||||||

// SERVES 4 //

4 eggs
approx. 1 litre sunflower
   or vegetable oil, for frying

CHICKEN CASING

400g minced chicken
2 garlic cloves, crushed to a paste,
   with a pinch of salt
2 tsp ground cumin
1 tbsp curry powder
¼ tsp ground white pepper
1 green or red chilli, deseeded
   and finely chopped
2 tbsp finely chopped coriander
1½ tsp salt

CRUMBED CASING

40g plain flour or oat flour
1 egg
splash milk
50g panko breadcrumbs
sea salt and freshly ground
   black pepper

1 / Put the eggs in a pan and cover with cold water. Bring to the boil, reduce the heat to a simmer and cook for 5 minutes. Drain and rinse under cold water to stop the eggs from cooking further. When cool enough to handle, peel.

2 / Put all the ingredients for the chicken in a bowl and mix well. Test the seasoning by frying up a little morsel of the mixture in a pan, then adjust to your liking. Remember if you're serving these cold, the salt will dull down. Divide the mixture into four meatballs.

3 / Season the flour with salt and pepper in one shallow bowl. Beat the eggs with the milk in another bowl and have the breadcrumbs spread out on a plate.

4 / Put a sheet of clingfilm on a work surface and lightly flour. Put one meatball in the centre and flour lightly, then place another sheet of clingfilm on top. Roll out the meat until large enough to encase an egg. Remove the top sheet of clingfilm.

5 / Dip the cooked egg in flour and dust off any excess. Place the egg in the centre of the meat. Bring up the sides of the clingfilm to encase it and smooth into a nice round. Dip each egg in flour, then beaten egg, followed by the breadcrumbs.

6 / Heat enough oil in a pan to come to about 3cm up the sides until it reaches about 170°C . If you don't have a thermometer, test the heat by dropping a crumb of bread into the hot oil; if it sizzles and turns golden but doesn't burn the oil is good to go. Cook the eggs a couple at a time for about 8–9 minutes, turning over as the outsides brown, until golden and crisp on the surface and done in the middle. Drain on kitchen paper and allow to cool completely before eating.

Who knows where Eggs Benedict really came from – all that matters is that it did. Thank you Benedict.

This muffin-free version is both quick and feels luxurious, a winning combination in our books.

Eggs Benedict omelette

||||||||||||||||||||||||||||||||||||||||||||||||||||||||||||||||||||||||||||||||||

// SERVES 1 //

1–2 rashers streaky bacon
  or slices ham
2 eggs
½ tsp Dijon mustard
pinch cayenne
few chives, snipped
small knob butter
small handful grated Gruyère
1 tbsp jarred
  hollandaise sauce
lemon wedge, to serve
sea salt and freshly ground
  black pepper

1 / Fry the bacon in a pan until nicely crisp or as done as you like. Chop up into small, bite-sized pieces.

2 / Crack the eggs into a bowl and whisk with the mustard, cayenne, chives and salt and pepper. Add the bacon pieces.

3 / Melt the butter in a pan over medium heat until foaming, add the eggs and move the pan around to spread them out evenly. When the omelette starts to firm up but still has a little raw egg on top, sprinkle over the cheese and dollop with hollandaise sauce. Use a spatula to gently fold half of the omelette over, into a half-moon. Cook for 2 minutes, until golden at the base, then flip over and cook the other side until golden. The omelette should be oozing with cheese and quite puffed on top.

4 / Remove from the heat and serve with a squeeze of lemon juice.

Protein + Oats = Proats

Sadly we can't claim credit for this winner of a word-mash, but we can claim credit for this awesome mix of goodness, all made overnight while you sleep for extra ease.

Ultimate chocolate proats

||||||||||||||||||||||||||||||||||||||||||||||||||||||||||||||||||||||||||||||||||||||||||||||

// SERVES 2 //

1 banana
100g porridge oats
2 tbsp honey
3 scoops chocolate whey
  protein powder
1 tbsp raw cocoa powder
  or cacao nibs
350–380ml almond milk
1 tbsp cashew or almond butter
  (optional)
fresh mixed berries, to serve

1 / Peel and slice the banana into a large bowl and roughly mash with a fork. Add the oats, honey, chocolate whey powder, cocoa powder and 350ml milk. Cover with clingfilm and leave in the fridge overnight.

2 / The next day, the mixture will have thickened so add a bit more milk. Serve with a dollop of cashew butter (if using) and fresh berries tumbled over the top.

The smell of homemade granola baking is a thing of beauty; layer up with your favourite yoghurt and fruit and you're on to a winner.

Homemade granola pots

||||||||||||||||||||||||||||||||||||||||||||||||||||||||||||||||||||||||||||||||||

// MAKES 8 SERVINGS //

100g coconut oil
6 tbsp maple syrup
2 tsp vanilla extract
300g jumbo rolled oats
300g mixed nuts (walnuts, pecans, almonds, cashews, hazelnuts)
100g ground almonds
100g mixed seeds (pumpkin, sunflower, sesame)
1 tbsp ground cinnamon
sea salt
200g dried fruit (prunes, figs, apricots, raisins, cherries, roughly chopped if large)

TO SERVE
fresh fruit of your choice
Greek yoghurt

1 / Preheat the oven to 190°C/Gas 5.

2 / Melt the coconut oil in a saucepan and stir in the maple syrup and vanilla extract.

3 / Put the oats in a large mixing bowl and add the mixed nuts (chop these in half if you like, but leave them quite chunky), ground almonds, seeds, ground cinnamon and a good pinch of salt. Stir everything together well. Pour the liquid ingredients into the bowl and stir until everything is well incorporated.

4 / Divide the mixture between 2 large baking trays and bake in the oven for 15 minutes. Take the trays out, give everything a stir, then switch the trays around and bake for a further 15 minutes, or until golden and crisp.

5 / Leave the granola to cool in the trays and, once cooled, mix in the chopped dried fruit.

6 / To serve, layer up the granola in a glass, alternating with spoonfuls of fresh Greek yoghurt and chopped fresh fruit. Store any remaining granola in an airtight container for up to 2 weeks.

These sound like they shouldn't work, but trust us - they really do! Perfect for brunch as well as taking in to the office, we like ours with lightly caramelised banana, but anything from berries to grilled bacon works a treat.

3-ingredient pancakes

||||||||||||||||||||||||||||||||||||||||||||||||||||||||||||||||||||||||||||||||||||||||||||||||||||||||||

// MAKES 6–8 //

2 small ripe bananas
2 heaped tbsp peanut butter
2 eggs, lightly beaten
coconut oil, for frying

TOPPING
1 tbsp coconut oil
1 small banana, sliced
pinch ground cinnamon
natural yoghurt
finely grated zest of 1 lime

1 / Mash the bananas with a fork until almost smooth. Add the peanut butter and mash together as much as you can to make a smooth mixture. Fold through the eggs until just combined.

2 / Heat the tablespoon of coconut oil in a small frying pan over medium heat. Slide the banana slices into the pan, sprinkle with cinnamon and let the banana brown and caramelise slightly at the edges, about 4–5 minutes. Flip over to brown the other side but don't overcook them to the point where they go too soft. Keep warm.

3 / Heat the oil in a frying pan over medium heat. Add spoonfuls of the pancake mixture to the pan and cook for 3–4 minutes, until the bottoms are golden brown. Flip over and continue to cook the other side for a further 3 minutes, or until cooked through. Continue cooking in batches until you run out of mixture.

4 / Serve the pancakes with the bananas toppled over, yoghurt dolloped on top and sprinkled with lime zest.

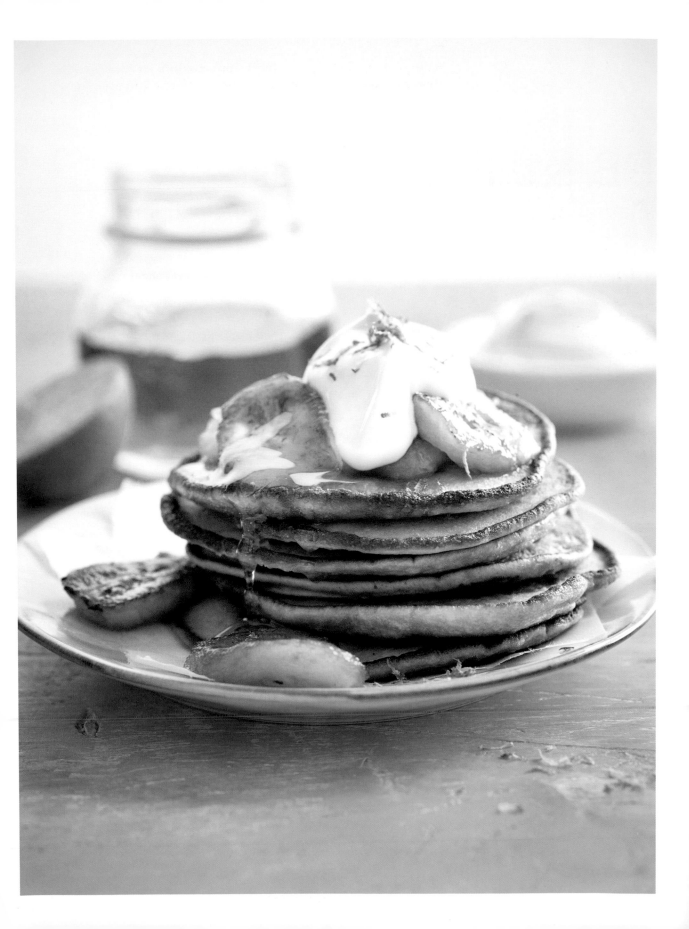

Behold the stuffed French Toast. It's actually a lot healthier than the ooziness might suggest, but definitely still packs one hell of a punch.

PB & J French Toast

|||||||||||||||||||||||||||||||||||||||||||||||||||||||||||||||||||||||||||||||||||||||||||||||

// MAKES 2 //

150g frozen raspberries
squeeze lemon juice
1 tbsp agave syrup or honey
2-3 tbsp smooth
   peanut butter
4 slices wholegrain bread
   (slightly stale is also good)
2 eggs
60ml almond milk
coconut oil

1 / Heat the raspberries, lemon juice and agave syrup or honey in a pan. Bring to a simmer and let the raspberries pop and bubble away for 5–8 minutes, until syrupy.

2 / Spread the peanut butter on two slices of bread and layer on the raspberry coulis. Top each slice of bread with the unbuttered bread to create two sandwiches.

3 / In a shallow bowl, beat the eggs and whisk together with the milk. Working with one at a time, dip the sandwiches into the egg mixture, turning to coat all over.

4 / Melt the coconut oil in a frying pan over medium heat and fry the soaked sandwiches for 4–6 minutes, or until brown, before flipping to cook the other side. Remove from the pan, cut in half and serve with extra raspberry coulis on the side.

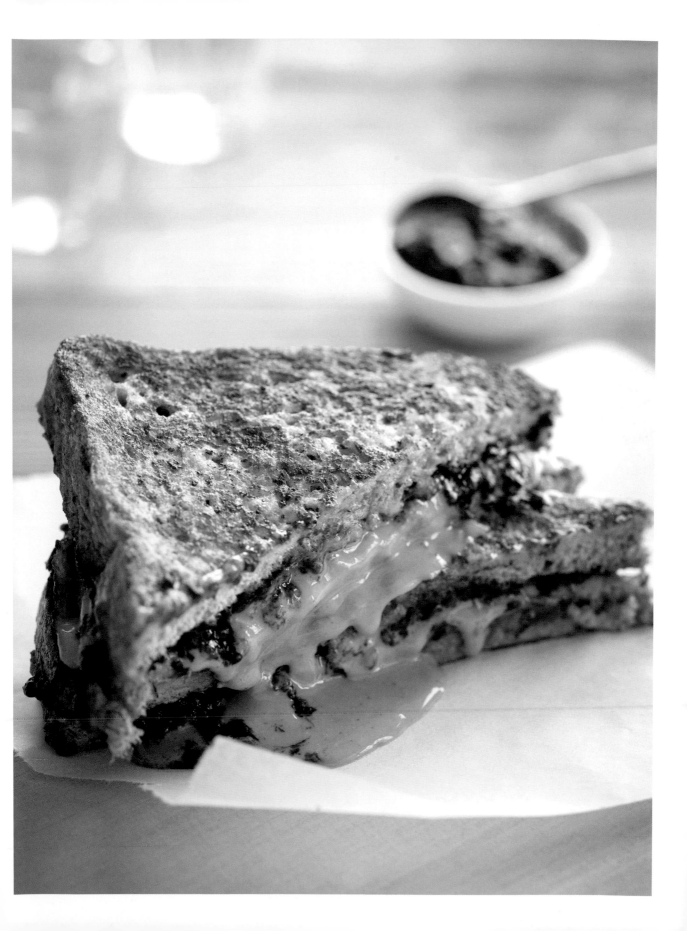

These are such a great thing to have a stash of, either at home as a grab-and-go breakfast, or to keep in your office for snack-time.

Honey fruit and oat bars

|||||||||||||||||||||||||||||||||||||||||||||||||||||||||||||||||||||||||||||||||||||||||||||

// MAKES 10–15 //

½ tsp ground cinnamon
200g jumbo oats
90g dried pitted dates, finely chopped
90g dried apricots, chopped
  (or raisins)
90g dried mango, chopped
50g chopped mixed nuts
  (almonds, cashews, hazelnuts)
100g unsalted butter, cubed
50g coconut sugar or raw sugar
140g honey
130ml fresh apple or orange juice
finely grated zest of 1 orange
pinch sea salt
120g mixed seeds (pumpkin,
  sunflower and sesame seeds)

1 / Preheat the oven to 180°C/Gas 4. Line a rectangular baking tray with baking parchment.

2 / Combine the cinnamon, oats, dried fruit and nuts in a bowl.

3 / Heat the butter, sugar, honey, fruit juice and orange zest in a saucepan over low heat. Stir occasionally until the butter has melted and the ingredients have combined. Take off the heat, add the cinnamon oats, dried fruit and nuts. Stir well, then mix in the salt and about 90g of the seeds.

4 / Spread the mixture into the prepared tin and flatten the surface with the back of a spoon. Sprinkle over the remaining seeds. Bake for 25–30 minutes, until golden brown.

5 / Let cool in the tin for at least 10 minutes before turning out and cutting into fingers. These will keep for up to 10 days in an airtight jar.

Lunch

‖‖‖

These light little bites are satisfyingly savoury; they also make great canapés for when you have friends over and are feeling fancy.

Tuna & white bean salad in little gem cups

||||||||||||||||||||||||||||||||||||||||||||||||||||||||||||||||||||||||||||||||||||||||||||||||||||||||||||||||||||||||

// MAKES 6 //

80g tinned tuna, drained
200g tinned cannellini beans
  or other white beans, well rinsed
  and drained
50g spring onions, finely sliced
2 tsp capers, roughly chopped
small handful parsley or basil leaves
¼ small red onion, very finely sliced
1 stalk celery, very finely diced
few shavings Parmesan
6 little gem leaves
sea salt and freshly ground
  black pepper

DRESSING
1 tbsp lemon juice
finely grated zest of ½ lemon
1 tbsp extra virgin olive oil

1 / Mix the dressing ingredients in a bowl. Break the tuna up into chunks into the bowl, add the remaining ingredients, apart from the little gem, and combine gently. Season to taste.

2 / Lay the lettuce leaves on a plate and divide up the bean salad evenly.

Our take on a French classic. Feel free to blitz it a bit at the end if you're after something a little thicker.

Caramelised red onion soup

||||||||||||||||||||||||||||||||||||||||||||||||||||||||||||||||||||||||||||||||

// SERVES 2 //

2 large red onions
1 tbsp red wine vinegar
knob unsalted butter
1 tbsp maple syrup
150g button mushrooms,
   finely sliced
2 sprigs thyme, leaves picked
   or 1 tsp dried thyme
700ml beef stock
60ml red wine
sea salt and freshly ground
   black pepper
1 tbsp cornflour, mixed into
   a paste with 1 tbsp water

1 / Slice the onions into wedges, place in a microwave-proof dish with the vinegar, butter and maple syrup and cover and cook on high for 7 minutes.

2 / Tip the onions into a large pan and cook over medium-low heat for 10 minutes, stirring, until the onions are caramelised. They will be very sweet and slightly darker in colour. Add the mushrooms and thyme and cook for about 5 minutes, until the mushrooms lose their moisture.

3 / Pour in the stock, wine and 250ml water, then bring to the boil. Let it boil away for 10–15 minutes.

4 / Stir through the cornflour paste and simmer for a couple of minutes to thicken. Season with salt and pepper to taste.

This has such a lovely balance of spice and warmth, with just the right amount of sweetness. A great lunch for the colder months, it's satisfying enough on its own, but as ever with soups a hunk of bread wouldn't go amiss.

Curried sweet potato & ginger soup

|||||||||||||||||||||||||||||||||||||||||||||||||||||||||||||||||||||||||||||||||||||||

// SERVES 2–3 //

30g unsalted butter

1 small carrot, finely chopped

1 small onion, finely chopped

thumbnail-sized piece fresh ginger, grated

2 tsp curry powder

500g sweet potatoes, peeled and chopped into small chunks

600ml chicken stock

3 tbsp crème fraîche, plus extra to serve (optional)

squeeze lemon juice, to serve

sea salt and freshly ground black pepper

1 / Melt the butter in a large pan over medium-low heat. Add the carrot and onion, along with a pinch of salt, cover and cook gently for 10 minutes, until softened but not browned and sweet.

2 / Add the ginger and curry powder and let them cook for a couple of minutes until aromatic. Tip in the sweet potatoes, cover and cook over medium heat, stirring occasionally, for 10 minutes. Pour in the stock, season with salt and pepper and bring to the boil. Simmer for 10 minutes, or until the potatoes are cooked through and soft.

3 / Add the crème fraîche and lemon juice, bring back to the boil quickly, then remove from the heat.

4 / Use a stick blender to liquidise. Taste and season as needed before serving with an extra dollop of crème fraîche, if you like.

Roasting the chickpeas gives them the most amazing crunchy texture. If you are short on time (or feeling a bit lazy) you can just chuck them in – either way this makes a super tasty and veg-packed lunch.

Superfood wrap

|||||||||||||||||||||||||||||||||||||||||||||||||||||||||||||||||||||||||||||||||||

// SERVES 2 //

210g tinned chickpeas, drained
2 tsp extra virgin olive oil
1 tsp ground cumin
½ tsp smoked paprika
few pinches ground allspice
pinch dried chilli
1 ripe avocado
juice of ½ lime
2 large wholemeal tortilla wraps
4–6 tenderstem broccoli, steamed
½ carrot, grated
handful watercress or rocket leaves
handful sprouted chia, radish
   or alfalfa
sea salt and freshly ground black
   pepper

TAHINI DRESSING
2 tbsp tahini
1 tbsp Greek yoghurt
1 tbsp lemon juice
1 tsp olive oil

1 / Preheat the oven to 200°C/Gas 6.

2 / Tip the chickpeas into a baking tray and toss them in the olive oil, cumin, paprika, allspice, chilli and season with salt and pepper. Roast in the oven for 20–25 minutes until starting to crisp. Shake the tray halfway through to prevent the chickpeas from catching.

3 / Meanwhile, combine the ingredients for the tahini dressing in a bowl and season with salt and pepper. Add 1–2 tablespoons cold water, if needed, to make a fluid consistency but not too runny.

4 / Cut the avocado in half and remove the stone. Scoop out the flesh, slice into large chunks and toss in a bowl with the lime juice. Warm the tortilla wraps according to the packet instructions. Pile on the broccoli, grated carrot, watercress, sprouts, avocado and the roasted chickpeas. Dollop over the dressing and wrap.

The flavours of this salad are unbelievably fresh and zingy – it also makes a great supper too if you're after something a little lighter.

Soy sesame chicken & cucumber salad

||||||||||||||||||||||||||||||||||||||||||||||||||||||||||||||||||||||||||||||||||||||||||||||||

// SERVES 2 //

1 tsp rice vinegar
1 tbsp soy sauce
1 tsp sesame oil
2 tbsp honey
1 red chilli, deseeded, plus extra
   sliced to serve
1 tbsp sesame seeds
juice of 1 lime
2 boneless, skinless chicken breasts
1 cucumber
iceberg or little gem lettuce
coriander leaves, to garnish
sea salt and freshly ground black
   pepper

DRESSING
juice of 1 lime
2 tsp sesame oil
2 tbsp soy sauce

1 / Make the marinade for the chicken by mixing together the rice vinegar, soy sauce, sesame oil, honey, chilli, lime juice and sesame seeds. Add the chicken breasts, coat all over and leave to marinate for at least 1 hour.

2 / When you are ready to cook, preheat a griddle pan over medium-high heat.

3 / Add the chicken and grill for about 8 minutes, until nicely charred on one side. Flip over and grill the other side until the chicken is cooked through.

4 / Remove from the heat and let sit for a moment on a chopping board while you prepare the vegetables and dressing.

5 / Mix the ingredients for the dressing together in a small bowl. Finely slice the cucumber into thins, if you have a mandoline all the better, otherwise just use a sharp knife. Shred the lettuce and arrange on plates with the cucumber.

6 / Slice the chicken into pieces and arrange on top of the salad. Spoon over the dressing, scatter with extra chilli and the coriander leaves and serve.

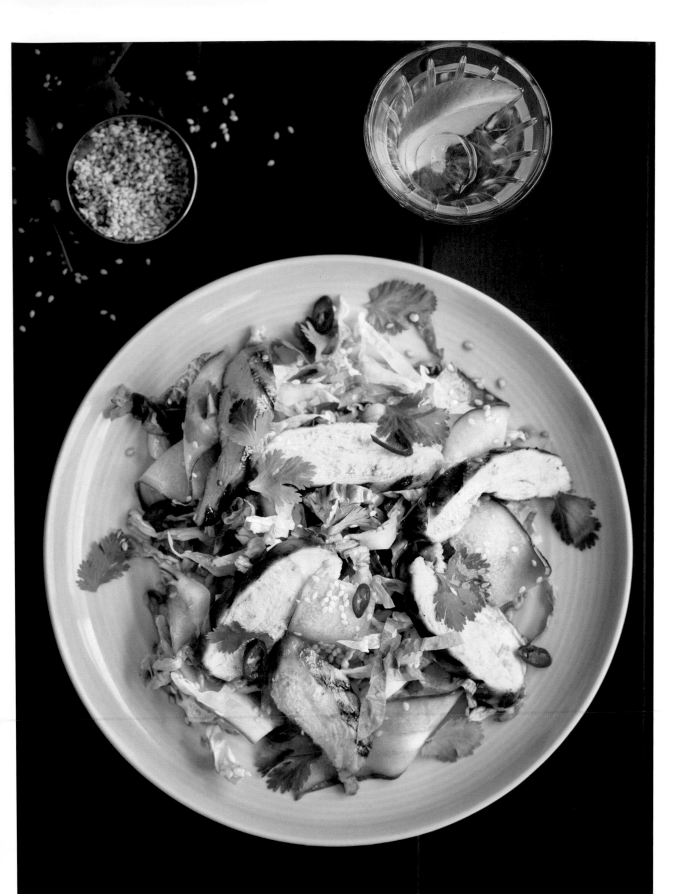

We've already mentioned our love of Mexican food, and this is another firm favourite. We cannot claim as to its authenticity, but it is certainly tasty! Don't be put off by what might seem like a long list of ingredients – a lot of them overlap for each component. And when you layer them up and beans meet rice meets salsa, all crowned with fresh guacamole, it is worth every second of your time.

Mexican layer bowl

‖‖

// SERVES 2–3 //

250g (about 1½ cups) cooked brown
   rice or quinoa
small handful coriander, chopped,
   plus extra for garnish
juice of ½ lime
2 large handfuls shredded cos lettuce
65g feta, crumbled
soured cream (optional)

SALSA
1 garlic clove, crushed
½ jalapeño chilli, finely chopped
1–2 tsp salt
¼ tsp ground cumin
juice of ½ lime
2 tbsp extra virgin olive oil
3 tomatoes, roughly diced
2 tbsp chopped coriander
sea salt and freshly ground
   black pepper

1 / Make the salsa. Bash the garlic, chilli, salt and cumin in a mortar and pestle. Add the lime juice and oil, then season and set aside.

2 / Put the tomatoes in a bowl and pour over the dressing. Mix well and add the coriander. Season to taste with salt and pepper. Chill for 10 minutes while you get on with the guacamole.

3 / Cut the avocado in half and remove the stone. Scoop the flesh into a bowl and mash roughly with the lime juice, coriander, tomato, garlic, onion, tabasco and cumin. Season with salt and pepper and chill until ready to serve.

4 / Mix the rice or quinoa with the coriander and lime juice. Set aside. (You can warm the rice or quinoa but it is equally good cold.)

TIP

This dish is a good opportunity to use up leftover rice, but do make sure to reheat the rice really thoroughly – you want it hotter than the sun – as it can be dangerous otherwise. The microwaveable pouches work well for this.

GUACAMOLE

1 ripe avocado

juice of ½ lime

small handful coriander, finely chopped

1 small tomato, deseeded and diced

1 small garlic clove, finely chopped

¼ red onion, very finely chopped

dash tabasco

½ tsp ground cumin

sea salt and freshly ground
  black pepper

BEANS

2 tbsp coconut oil or olive oil

1 small onion, diced

2 garlic cloves, finely chopped

pinch of salt

90g tinned sweetcorn kernels, drained

220g tinned cooked black beans,
  rinsed and drained

2 medium tomatoes, diced

pinch cayenne

1 tsp dried oregano

2 tbsp tomato purée

small handful coriander, chopped

5 / Now prepare the beans. Heat the oil in a pan and fry the onion and garlic along with a pinch of salt for 5–6 minutes, until the onion is softened but not browned. Add the sweetcorn, black beans and tomatoes, and stir well. Add the cayenne, oregano and tomato purée. Let the mixture simmer for 10–12 minutes to allow the tomatoes to break down.

6 / When you are ready to serve, divide the rice between bowls, top each with some lettuce, a couple of scoops of the black bean and corn, the salsa, feta and guacamole. Garnish with chopped spring onions and coriander, and a good dollop of soured cream, if you like.

Sushi is such a great lunch option – easy, healthy, high-protein – and making your own is actually remarkably simple. We use cling film to make ours which works really well, so don't worry if you don't have a sushi mat. Experiment with your fillings too – as well as the options below try cooked prawns, baby corn or a little roast chicken.

Easy-peasy sushi

||||||||||||||||||||||||||||||||||||||||||||||||||||||||||||||||||||||||||||||||||

// MAKES 36 //

210g short-grain rice or Japanese
  sushi rice
3 tbsp rice wine vinegar
1½ tbsp unrefined sugar
2 tsp salt
6 nori seaweed sheets
Japanese soy sauce, for dipping

OPTIONAL FILLINGS
(CHOOSE FROM ANY)
raw salmon (skin and bones removed)
  or smoked salmon, cut into strips
avocado, destoned and flesh
  cut into strips
cucumber, cut into finger-width strips
tinned tuna
white crabmeat
red pepper, cut into strips

1 / Rinse the rice and drain well. Put in a pan with 250ml water and bring to the boil. Reduce the heat to low, cover with the lid and cook for 12 minutes. Remove from the heat and let it stand for 15 minutes, without taking off the lid. Meanwhile, heat the rice wine vinegar, sugar and salt in a small pan and stir to dissolve. Take off the heat and let it cool briefly.

2 / When the rice is done, stir the vinegar-sugar mixture through, using a fork. Spread out over a plate and let it sit while you prepare the fillings. The rice can be made 48 hours in advance and stored in the fridge with clingfilm over it.

3 / Lay a nori sheet on a sheet of clingfilm, shiny side down. Place a handful of rice on top and pat it down until the rice covers the nori, leaving about a 5cm-wide border.

4 / Lay your chosen fillings, a few strips only, along the bottom edge of the rice in a line. Starting with the edge closest to you, roll up the clingfilm and nori together as tightly as possible, enclosing the filling. Pull out the clingfilm as you roll so that it doesn't get caught in the sushi roll. When you get to the border at the top edge, dab the nori with a little water, then roll up to seal. Repeat with the remaining nori sheets, rice and fillings.

5 / Chill, join side down, for 15 minutes before serving.

6 / To serve, slice the rolls crosswise into 6 pieces and serve with soy sauce for dipping on the side.

This is such a satisfying lunch – warm and filling, make up a batch on Sunday afternoon and bring the rest in to work. Add a pouch of microwaveable rice to bulk it up for a hearty supper.

Chicken korma soup

||||||||||||||||||||||||||||||||||||||||||||||||||||||||||||||||||||||||||||||||||||

// SERVES 2–3 //

1 tbsp coconut oil
1 medium onion, finely chopped
1½ celery stalks, finely chopped
small bunch coriander, stalks chopped and leaves reserved (optional)
2 garlic cloves
thumbnail-sized piece fresh ginger, grated
½ tsp turmeric
2 tbsp korma curry paste
1 × 400g tin coconut cream
2 handfuls cashew nuts, plus extra to serve
500ml vegetable or chicken stock
2 chicken breast fillets, sliced
handful green beans
natural yoghurt, to serve
sea salt and freshly ground black pepper

1 / Heat the oil in a pan, add the onion, celery and coriander stalks, if using, and cook over medium heat for 10–15 minutes, until softened and sweet. Add the garlic, ginger, turmeric and curry paste, then continue to cook for another 5 minutes. Pour in the coconut cream and add the cashews. Bring to the boil, reduce the heat and simmer for 10 minutes.

2 / Use a stick blender to blend the soup to a purée. Drop in the chicken slices and beans and simmer gently for 10 minutes until the chicken is cooked through. Season to taste with salt and pepper.

3 / Serve ladled into soup bowls with a few extra cashew nuts on top and some coriander leaves if you like. A swirl of yoghurt to cool down the soup also goes down a treat.

LLOYD'S TIP

For a vegetarian version, swap the chicken with cooked chickpeas.

This works with pretty much anything; below is our favourite combination, but you can fill your jar with everything from pasta and pesto to courgetti and cream cheese – the point (and the fun) is in the shake.

Shake-it-jar salad

||||||||||||||||||||||||||||||||||||||||||||||||||||||||||||||||||||||||||||||||||||||||||||||

// SERVES 2 //

¼ medium butternut squash,
 peeled and cut into 2cm cubes
160g cooked chickpeas
 (tinned are fine)
4–5 cherry tomatoes
12 olives
100g feta, cubed
little gem lettuce leaves,
 torn into bite-sized pieces
2 handfuls rocket leaves
 or watercress
mixed seeds and nuts such as
 sesame seeds, sunflower or
 pumpkin seeds, almonds
 and walnuts

DRESSING (APPROX. 100ML)
3 tbsp extra virgin olive oil
finely grated zest and juice of
 ½ lemon
1 tsp agave syrup
sea salt and freshly ground
 black pepper

1 / Have two Mason jars ready to fill with your salad ingredients.

2 / Start with the heaviest ingredients and dressing at the bottom so the leaves have no chance of getting soggy.

3 / First, prepare the butternut squash by putting in a bowl with water to come about 2cm up the sides of the bowl. Steam in the microwave for 5–10 minutes, on high, until fork-tender. Drain well and allow to cool completely.

4 / Mix together the ingredients for the dressing in a small bowl and add about 1–2 tablespoons dressing per jar. (The remaining dressing can be saved for other salads.) Divide the chickpeas and cherry tomatoes between the jars, then layer with the butternut squash cubes followed by the olives. Screw on the lids and pop into the fridge until ready to eat. (It will last like this for a couple of days in the fridge.)

5 / Just before eating, add the feta cubes, little gem, rocket, seeds and nuts, and shake it all up.

MAX'S TIPS

Adding tarragon leaves or basil to the dressing brightens the salad.

Try a mix of cooked beans instead of the chickpeas; black beans or white beans work especially well. Basically any combination of fresh vegetables you like can go in this salad – cooked beetroot and cucumber are excellent additions too.

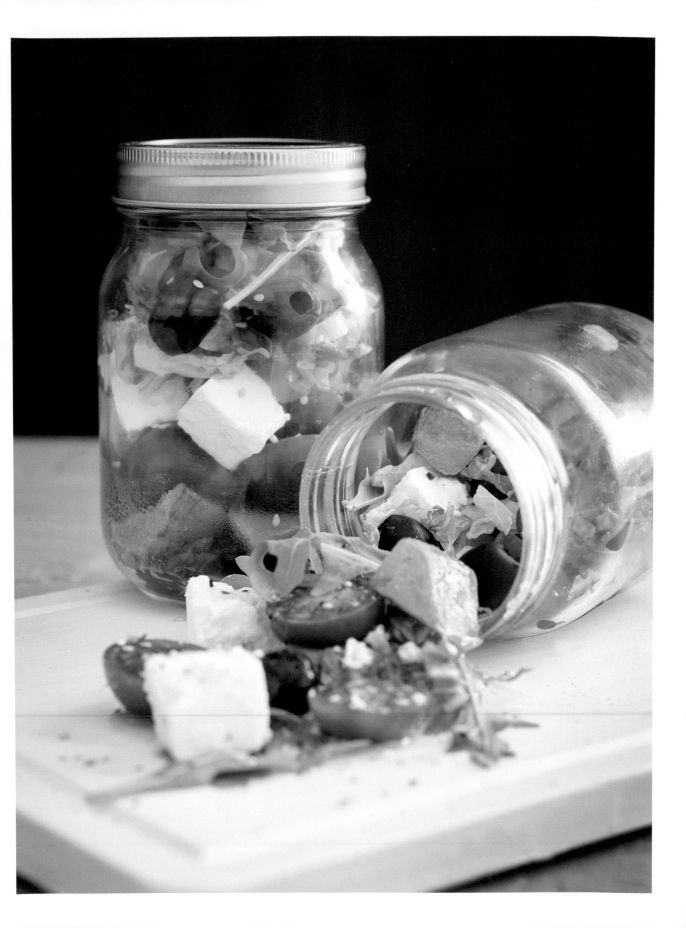

A fresh take on two humble classics, the potato salad and egg salad; this is amazing on its own, and equally good piled high on a plate of green leaves or on a slice of toasted ciabatta.

Roast sweet potato & egg salad

|||||||||||||||||||||||||||||||||||||||||||||||||||||||||||||||||||||||||||||||||||||||||||||

// SERVES 4 //

1 tsp coconut oil, for frying
1 medium sweet potato, peeled
  and cut into 1cm cubes
pinch cayenne
1–2 tsp olive oil
4 lean bacon strips (optional)
6 eggs
2 small shallots, finely chopped
small bunch chives, snipped
1 sprig dill, chopped
1 celery stalk, sliced
3–4 tbsp good-quality mayonnaise
2 tsp white wine vinegar
toasted flaked almonds
sea salt and freshly ground
  black pepper

1 / Preheat the oven to 200°C/Gas 6.

2 / Scatter the sweet potato on a baking tray and toss with the cayenne, salt and pepper. Drizzle with the oil. Cover with foil and bake for 20 minutes. Take off the foil and return to the oven to bake for a further 15 minutes, or until soft and golden at the edges. Allow to cool.

3 / If using bacon, place on a baking tray lined with baking parchment and bake in the oven for 10–12 minutes, until crisp.

4 / Put the eggs in a pan with fresh water to cover. Bring to the boil over high heat, reduce the heat to a simmer and cook for 4–5 minutes. Take off the heat and rinse under cold, running water to stop the eggs from cooking further. Peel them as soon as they are cold enough to handle.

5 / Roughly cut the eggs into quarters and put them in a bowl. Combine with the shallots, chives, dill and celery, and tear the bacon into pieces, if using. Add the sweet potato, mayonnaise and vinegar, and fold everything together gently so as not to break the eggs up too much. Season to taste with salt and pepper and serve with the flaked almonds scattered on top.

These are equally good cold too. And don't be afraid to use good-quality tinned salmon if you are pressed for time, or tuna. For a more substantial meal, try serving them with a poached or fried egg.

Salmon & quinoa bites

||||||||||||||||||||||||||||||||||||||||||||||||||||||||||||||||||||||||||||||||||||||||||

// MAKES 20 //

200g cooked red, white or
  mixed quinoa
220g cooked skinless salmon fillet,
  roughly flaked
½ red onion, finely chopped
1 plump garlic clove, finely crushed
  to a paste
small bunch dill, finely chopped
finely grated zest of 1 lemon
2 tbsp oat flour or ground almonds
2 eggs
4 tbsp coarse polenta
1 tbsp coconut oil or olive oil
lemon wedges, to serve
sea salt and freshly ground
  black pepper

DILL YOGHURT
60g Greek yoghurt
½ garlic clove, crushed to a paste
1 dill sprig, finely chopped

1 / Put the quinoa, salmon, onion, garlic, dill, lemon zest, oat flour or ground almonds in a bowl. Mix well and season with salt and pepper. Beat the eggs and add to the bowl too, then mix again. Divide the mixture up and roll into golfballs. Squash lightly into a small cake. If you have time, chill the cakes for 15–20 minutes to help them firm up.

2 / Mix the yoghurt with the garlic, 1 tablespoon cold water and the dill. Season to taste.

3 / When you are ready to cook, put the polenta on a plate and season with salt and pepper. Transfer the fishcakes to the plate with the polenta and pat all over.

4 / Heat the oil in a frying pan over medium heat. Add the fishcakes, a few at the time, and fry for about 8 minutes, letting the bottom form a nice crust, turning until the coating is crisp and brown and the cakes are piping hot in the middle.

5 / Serve immediately with the yoghurt, lemon wedges for squeezing and some crisp green leaves.

Cauliflower cheese in fritter form, these taste indulgent but are actually remarkably light. The sharpness of the dijon mustard cuts through the cheese, and paired with some peppery rocket they make a great lunch.

Cheesy cauliflower fritters

||||||||||||||||||||||||||||||||||||||||||||||||||||||||||||||||||||||||||||||||||||

// MAKES 10–12 //

560g cauliflower florets,
    cut into small 1cm pieces
2 eggs
90g plain flour
110g mature Cheddar cheese,
    grated
1 tbsp Dijon mustard
generous pinch cayenne
splash or 2 of milk
1 tbsp olive oil
sea salt and freshly ground
    black pepper
Greek yoghurt or soured cream,
    to serve

1 / Bring a pan of water to the boil and blanch the cauliflower for 5–6 minutes, until tender to bite. Drain well and set aside.

2 / Beat the eggs in a large bowl, add the flour, cheese, mustard and cayenne and season with salt and pepper. Add a splash of milk to loosen the batter. Check the mixture for seasoning by frying up a small amount in a pan, then adjusting the seasoning to taste. Add the cauliflower pieces to the batter.

3 / Heat the oil in a frying pan over medium-high heat. Add tablespoonfuls of the batter, reduce the heat to medium and cook the fritters for 3–4 minutes until golden brown. (You may need to cook them in batches to prevent overcrowding the pan.) Only flip over once a nice crust has formed, then cook the other side until golden. Remove to kitchen paper to drain.

4 / Serve hot, with soured cream or yoghurt on the side.

MAX'S TIP:

To make a super-quick relish to go on the side, halve some cherry tomatoes, add some finely chopped red onion, chives and a squeeze of lemon.

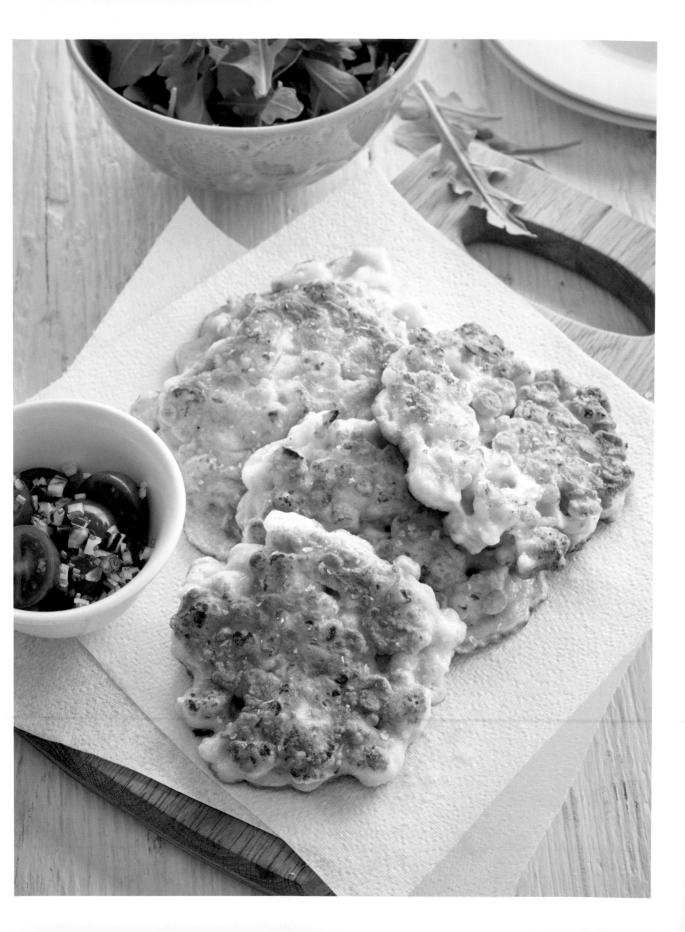

Created in the 1950s this is proper retro, and you'd be forgiven if the very name conjures up thoughts of old school black forest gateau and cheese cubes served on sticks. But the mix of mayo and yoghurt keeps this light, and it is a great way to use up leftover roast-chicken (see page 108). Pile on some salad leaves, scoop up with wholegrain toast or stuff into some pitta – you really can't go wrong!

Coronation chicken

|||||||||||||||||||||||||||||||||||||||||||||||||||||||||||||||||||||||||||||||||||||||

// SERVES 2 //

80g good-quality mayonnaise

80g natural yoghurt

1 tbsp mango chutney

2–3 tsp Madras curry powder, to taste

1 tsp Worcestershire sauce

1 celery stalk, sliced

2 leftover cold, cooked chicken breasts (about 200g), shredded into bite-sized pieces

25g fresh grapes, halved (or use raisins)

sea salt and freshly ground black pepper

TO SERVE

small bunch coriander, roughly chopped

lemon wedges

2 tbsp toasted flaked almonds

1 / In a bowl, combine the mayonnaise, yoghurt, chutney, curry powder and Worcestershire sauce. Season to taste. Add the celery, chicken and grapes, and gently fold together.

2 / Put in the fridge for at least 2 hours for the flavours to come together.

3 / Just before serving, fold through most of the coriander. Serve with a few lemon wedges for squeezing and the toasted almonds and remaining coriander sprinkled over the top.

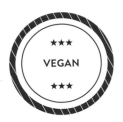

This is a great recipe to use up whatever veg you have leftover in your fridge – just vary the cooking times accordingly. The pesto is amazing without having to add the parmesan (the nuts add thickness and texture) so leave it out if you want to keep things vegan. Great on its own as a light lunch, the veggies and pesto are awesome stirred through some quinoa or pasta shapes too.

Roast vegetables & Brazil nut pesto

||||||||||||||||||||||||||||||||||||||||||||||||||||||||||||||||||||||||||||||||||||

// SERVES 4 //

1 small aubergine, diced into 2cm chunks

1 courgette, sliced into 2cm slices and cut into half-moons

1 red pepper, cut into quarters lengthwise, then halved widthwise

1 yellow pepper, cut into quarters lengthwise, then halved widthwise

¼ butternut squash, cut into 1cm cubes (no need to peel)

1 red onion, peeled and chopped into 6 wedges

4 whole garlic cloves (unpeeled)

generous glug olive oil

2 tbsp balsamic vinegar

1 large handful cherry tomatoes

sea salt and freshly ground black pepper

BRAZIL NUT PESTO

50g fresh basil leaves

20g Brazil nuts, roughly chopped

1 garlic clove, roughly chopped

20g Parmesan cheese, finely grated (optional)

zest of ½ lemon

4 tbsp extra virgin olive oil

1 tbsp lemon juice

1 / Preheat the oven to 190°C/Gas 5.

2 / Put all the prepared vegetables (except the cherry tomatoes) and garlic cloves into a large baking tray and drizzle with plenty of olive oil and the balsamic vinegar. Season well with salt and pepper.

3 / Put the tray in the oven and roast for 20 minutes. Remove from the oven and stir everything around. Add the cherry tomatoes, stir briefly again to coat them in the oil and return to the oven for a further 15–20 minutes, until all the vegetables are tender and beginning to brown.

4 / Meanwhile, make the pesto. Put all the ingredients into the small bowl of a food processor or a mini chopper and blitz to form a smooth pesto. Taste and season with salt and pepper.

5 / Once the veg are cooked, squeeze the garlic flesh out of the skins and stir it through the rest of the vegetables. Serve the roasted vegetables with the pesto to spoon over.

Dinner

||||||||||||||||||||||||||||||||||||||||||||||||||||

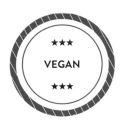

This is one of our favourite inventions. It might sound a little out there, but trust us on this – it is so moreish and the combination of slightly sweet (cinnamon) and savoury (tahini and garlic) really hits the spot. Steeping the red onions in lemon juice and hot water takes away the bitterness and turns them the most amazingly vibrant colour.

Moroccan pizza

||||||||||||||||||||||||||||||||||||||||||||||||||||||||||||||||||||||||||||||||||||||||||||

// SERVES 2 //

¼ cauliflower head, broken into florets
2 garlic cloves, crushed
200g tinned chickpeas, rinsed and
    drained
1 tsp smoked paprika
2 tsp ground cumin
1 tbsp olive oil
1 sweet potato, peeled and
    cut into small cubes
2 tbsp almond milk
pinch ground cinnamon
½ red onion, thinly sliced
juice of ½ lemon
2 large wholemeal tortilla wraps
sea salt and freshly ground
    black pepper

TAHINI SAUCE
60ml tahini
1 garlic clove, finely crushed
juice of 1 lemon

1 / Preheat the oven to 200°C/Gas 6.

2 / Scatter the cauliflower florets in a baking tray. Toss with the garlic, chickpeas, paprika, cumin and olive oil. Season with salt and pepper, then roast in the oven for 25–30 minutes, or until the cauliflower is golden brown.

3 / Meanwhile, put the sweet potato in a pan and cover with water. Bring to the boil and simmer until fork-tender. Remove from the heat, drain and return the sweet potato to the pan. Add the milk, cinnamon and season to taste. Mash until smooth and combined, adding a splash more milk if needed. Set aside.

4 / Put the red onion in a bowl with the lemon juice and let steep for 10 minutes.

5 / Mix the tahini with the garlic and lemon juice, and add 2–3 tablespoons warm water to make a fluid sauce. Season to taste.

6 / When ready to serve, take the tortilla wraps and spread them generously with the sweet potato mash. Top with the cauliflower and chickpeas. Drain the onions and sprinkle over the top. Serve drizzled with tahini sauce.

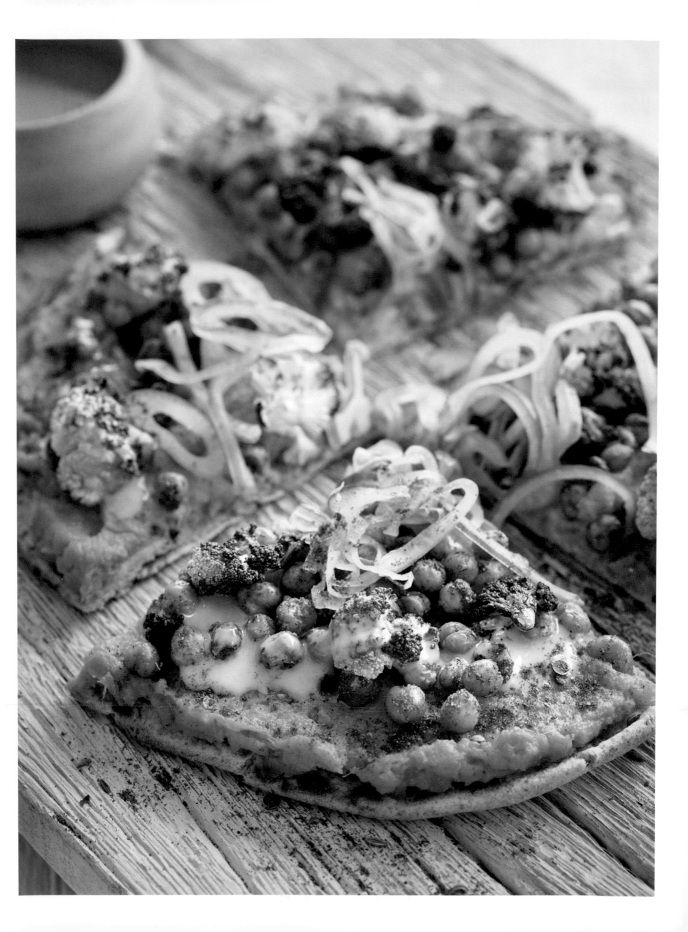

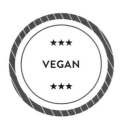

★★★

VEGAN

★★★

Don't be put off by the list of ingredients here – it might seem long, but most will either be things you have to hand in your store cupboard already, or will be worth buying for the future (see our note on Stocking Up, page 43). You'd never guess that there wasn't meat in this dish, and it makes the perfect meal to serve for vegans, veggies and die-hard carnivores alike.

Chilli no-carne

||||||||||||||||||||||||||||||||||||||||||||||||||||||||||||||||||||||||||||||||||||||||||||||||||

// SERVES 4 //

1 tbsp coconut oil, for frying

1 large onion, finely chopped

3 garlic cloves, finely chopped

3 tsp ground cumin

2 tsp ground allspice

2 tsp smoked paprika

1 cinnamon stick or 2 tsp ground cinnamon

2 bay leaves

1 tbsp chopped fresh oregano or 2 tsp dried oregano

1 medium courgette, diced

170g brown mushrooms, cut into slightly larger dice than the courgette

1 ancho chilli in sauce or 1 red chilli, split in half lengthways and deseeded

1 × 400g tin chopped tomatoes

1 tbsp cider or balsamic vinegar

1 tbsp maple syrup

1 tbsp tomato ketchup

50g dark chocolate (at least 70 per cent cocoa solids), roughly chopped

370ml vegetable stock

1 × 400g tin borlotti beans or black beans, rinsed and drained

sea salt and freshly ground black pepper

1 / Heat the oil in a large casserole pan, add the onion and a pinch of salt. Allow to cook over low heat, covered, for 10 minutes, stirring occasionally, until softened but not brown.

2 / Add the garlic along with the spices, bay leaves and oregano. Stir for 2 minutes, to let the spices become aromatic, then add the courgette. Cook for 5 minutes, until slightly softened, then add the mushrooms and fry for 5 more minutes until browned.

3 / Add the chilli, tomatoes, vinegar, maple syrup, ketchup and chocolate. Bring to the boil, stirring to melt the chocolate,

4 / Add the vegetable stock and beans, and bring back to the boil. Lower the heat to a simmer, season with salt and pepper, partially cover with a lid, then allow to cook for 40–50 minutes, until the courgette is tender.

5 / Serve in bowls over rice or in tortillas, with your choice of garnishes.

TO SERVE

cooked brown rice or soft tortillas / avocado slices / shredded cabbage / sliced radishes / coriander leaves / lime wedges

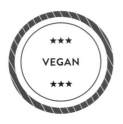

★★★

VEGAN

★★★

The yearly Halloween dilemma... what to do with the leftover innards of your lantern masterpiece? Well panic no more because this is a great option – warming and spicy, serve on its own or with some brown basmati rice and naan.

Pumpkin & cauliflower curry

||||||||||||||||||||||||||||||||||||||||||||||||||||||||||||||||||||||||||||||||

// SERVES 4–6 //

2 tbsp rapeseed or olive oil

1 large onion, finely chopped

2 large garlic cloves, finely chopped

½ red chilli, finely chopped

1 tbsp ground coriander

2 tsp ground cumin

2 tsp garam masala

400ml vegetable stock

1 x 400ml tin coconut milk

1 x 400g tin chopped tomatoes

½ pumpkin or 1 small butternut squash, peeled and cut into 2cm chunks (about 600g total weight)

1 small head cauliflower, chopped into large florets

150g red lentils

200g spinach

sea salt and freshly ground black pepper

1 / Heat the oil in a large pan and cook the onion over a low–medium heat for about 8 minutes, until softened and translucent. Add the garlic, chilli and spices and cook for another 2 minutes.

2 / Pour in the vegetable stock, coconut milk and the tinned tomatoes and add the pumpkin or butternut chunks. Bring to the boil, then let it bubble away for 15 minutes.

3 / Add the cauliflower florets and lentils and simmer for a further 10–15 minutes, until the cauliflower and pumpkin are cooked and the lentils have absorbed most of the excess to liquid to create a rich, thick sauce.

4 / Take the pan off the heat and stir through the spinach – there's no need to cook this as it will wilt in the heat of the curry. Season really well with salt and pepper and serve.

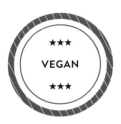

We promised you no BS in this book, so when we say *the best* vegan burger we mean the best. Easily doubled, these are great cooked on the BBQ, baked in the oven or on the hob. The celeriac slaw is a revelation too, and if you can't find a celeriac, red or white cabbage work equally well.

The best vegan burger

|||||||||||||||||||||||||||||||||||||||||||||||||||||||||||||||||||||||||||||||||||||||

// SERVES 2 //

THE BURGER

3 spring onions
1 red pepper, roughly chopped
4 garlic cloves
1 tsp smoked paprika
2 tsp ground cumin
1 tsp salt
handful cashews
handful pumpkin seeds
1 x 400g tin butter beans or haricot
  beans, rinsed and drained
1 tsp olive oil
freshly ground black pepper

CELERIAC SLAW

½ celeriac, grated
1 tbsp coconut yoghurt
1 tsp tamari
1 tbsp sesame oil
zest and juice of ½ lime

TO SERVE

2 soft vegan burger buns
lettuce or rocket leaves
sliced gherkins
sliced tomato

1 / Put the spring onions, pepper and garlic in a food processor and blend until chopped. Add the paprika, cumin, salt, cashews and seeds and pulse-blend until the mixture becomes the texture of breadcrumbs. Transfer to a bowl.

2 / Put the beans and oil in the food processor, and pulse with 2 teaspoons of cold water until smooth. Mix this into the nut and pepper mixture. Season to taste with salt and pepper.

3 / Roll the mix into large patties and chill in the fridge for at least 10 minutes.

4 / Meanwhile, make the slaw by mixing the ingredients together. Season to taste.

5 / To cook the burgers, heat a large pan over medium heat. Fry the burgers for 8 minutes on each side, or until golden and hot all the way through.

6 / Split the burger buns and add the slaw, lettuce, gherkins, tomato and a burger. Add the bun top and serve.

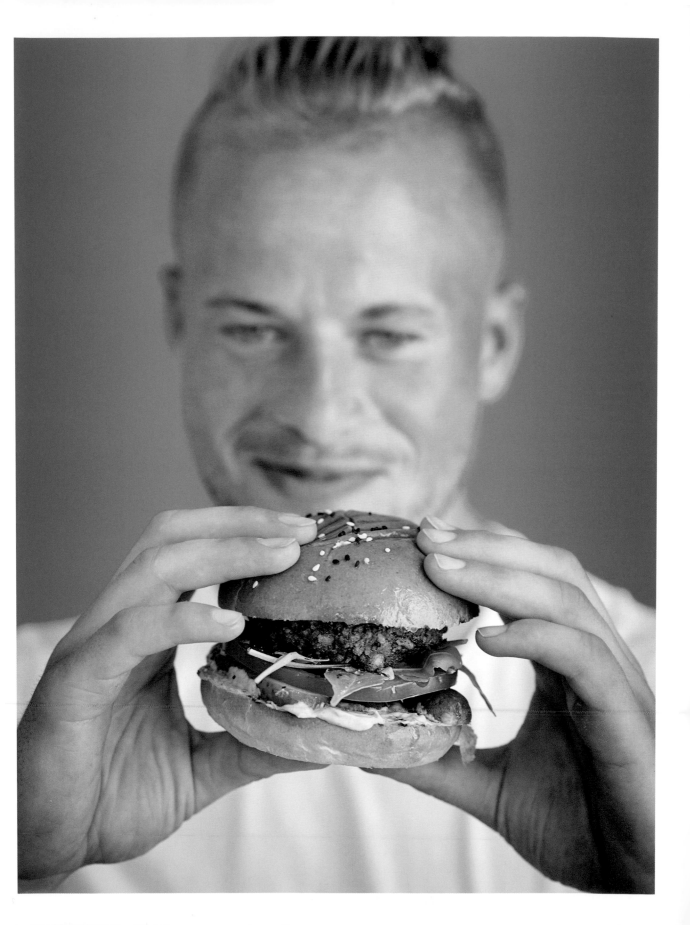

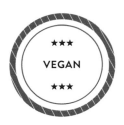

You might already be converted to tofu, still on the fence, or have no idea how to even say it; hopefully this dish might be the one to convert you! Tofu is pretty bland on its own but acts like a sponge to soak up flavours, making it particularly delicious in dishes that use tamarai or soy sauce, as this one does; marinating is definitely worth the effort here.

Marinated tofu stir-fry

|||||||||||||||||||||||||||||||||||||||||||||||||||||||||||||||||||||||||||||||||||||||

// SERVES 2 //

2 tbsp sunflower oil
3 tbsp soy sauce
2 tbsp rice wine
2 tbsp fish sauce
1 x 200g block firm tofu,
   cut into 2.5cm cubes
2 garlic cloves, finely chopped
thumb-sized piece ginger,
   peeled and sliced into
   fine matchsticks
1 small aubergine, cubed
100g baby corn
100g sugar snap peas
1 small red chilli, deseeded
   and sliced
large pinch ground white pepper
brown rice, to serve
handful coriander, chopped
black sesame seeds, to garnish
   (optional)
sea salt

1 / Whisk 1 tablespoon each of the soy sauce, rice wine and fish sauce and pour over the tofu cubes. Leave to marinate for 30 minutes to an hour; while marinating preheat your oven to 200°C/Gas 6. When you are ready, cover the tofu in some foil and bake in the oven for 20 minutes, turning occasionally.

2 / Heat the oil in a frying pan or wok. Add the garlic and ginger to the pan and fry for 2 minutes, until aromatic. Add the aubergine and stir-fry for 4–5 minutes, until slightly browned. Add the corn, sugar snap peas, chilli, remaining soy sauce, rice wine and fish sauce, and stir-fry for 3 more minutes. Add 2 tablespoons of water and continue to stir-fry until the water has evaporated. Add the pepper, season with extra salt to taste if needed.

3 / Serve over freshly cooked brown rice, scattered with coriander leaves and black sesame seeds, if using.

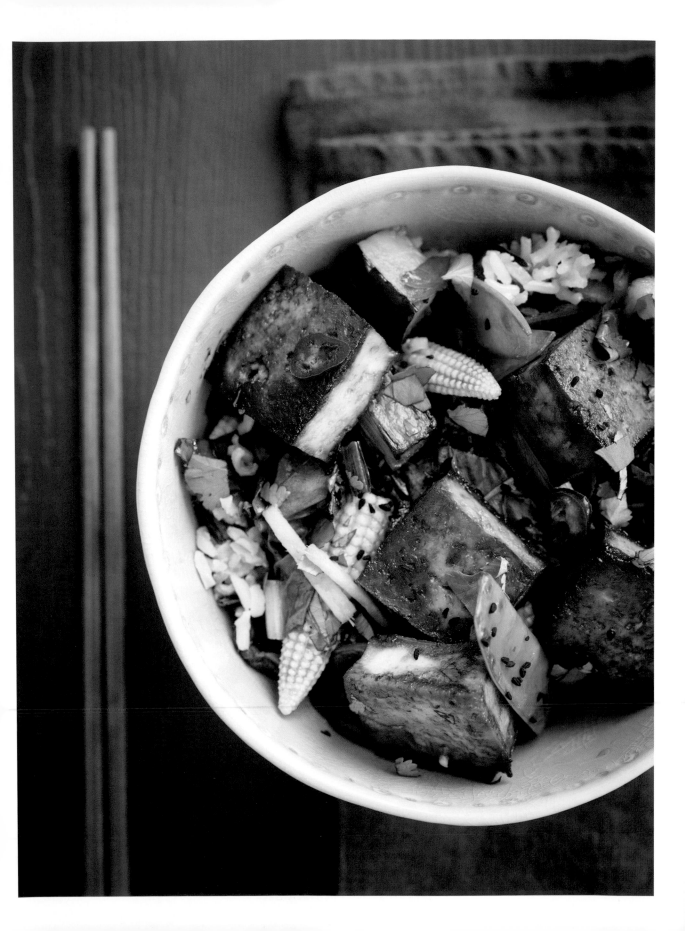

Full of vibrant flavours and a real chilli kick, this is such a comforting dish and perfect for when you're feeling a little under the weather. Feel free to swap the beef for chicken, tofu or prawns, or the rice noodles for egg noodles if that's what you have to hand.

Beef ramen

||||||||||||||||||||||||||||||||||||||||||||||||||||||||||||||||||||||||||||||||||||

// SERVES 4 //

3 garlic cloves, roughly chopped
2.5cm piece ginger, peeled and
   chopped, plus 2 extra large slices
250g beef sirloin or rump steaks
   (frying steaks are best)
1 long red chilli
4 tbsp soy sauce
2 tbsp sesame oil
1 tbsp rice wine vinegar
   or white vinegar
1½ tsp brown sugar
2 eggs
125g baby corn
2 spring onions, sliced
1.5 litres beef or chicken stock
3 tbsp fish sauce
250g rice noodles
coriander leaves, to garnish
white and black **sesame seeds**,
   to garnish
sea salt and freshly ground
   black pepper

1 / Put the garlic and ginger in a food processor and blitz to a fine paste. Tip into a bowl and combine with the beef, chilli and 2 tablespoons of the soy sauce. Add 1 tablespoon of the sesame oil, the vinegar and sugar and leave to marinate for 30 minutes.

2 / Put the eggs in a pan and cover with cold water. Bring to the boil and simmer for 4 minutes, drain and run under cold water. Peel as soon as the eggs are cool enough to handle and set aside.

3 / Heat a pan over high heat and sear the beef for 2–3 minutes each side, until cooked to your liking. Take off the heat and slice up.

4 / In a large, deep pan, heat the remaining sesame oil and fry the corn, spring onions and sliced ginger over high heat for 2–3 minutes. Add the stock and bring to the boil. Add the remaining soy and fish sauce, and season to taste with salt and pepper. Add the noodles and simmer for 4–5 minutes, until the noodles are cooked.

5 / Ladle the soup and noodles between bowls and serve with the beef and half an egg on top. Finally, garnish with coriander leaves and sesame seeds, and serve.

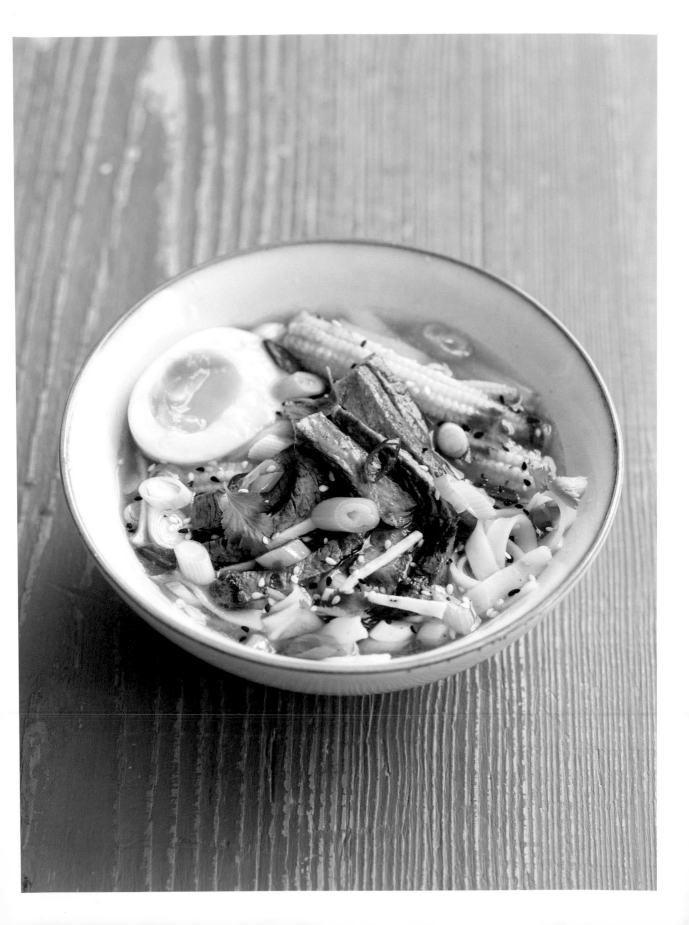

This is a great way to use up any leftover Brazil nut pesto (page 79), or you can make the classic version here. That said if you do go for shop-bought stuff we won't hold it against you (for long...). The focus here is on the perfectly cooked salmon; for what is a very simple dish to put together it is surprisingly elegant.

Pesto salmon parcels

||||||||||||||||||||||||||||||||||||||||||||||||||||||||||||||||||||||||||||||||||||||||

// SERVES 2 //

2 × 150g salmon fillets
zest of ½ lemon
2 pinches dried chilli flakes
4–6 tenderstem broccoli stems
extra virgin olive oil
sea salt and freshly ground
   black pepper

BASIL PINE NUT PESTO
2 handfuls basil leaves
2 tbsp pine nuts
1 garlic clove, roughly chopped
50–70ml olive oil
30g pecorino or Parmesan,
   finely grated

1 / Preheat the oven to 200°C/Gas 6. Make the pesto by blitzing the ingredients in a mini food processor, adding enough oil to get a nice pourable consistency. Season with salt and pepper to taste.

2 / Season the salmon fillets with salt and pepper. Cut two large squares of foil (about 50cm). Place one piece of salmon on each foil square. Grate over the lemon zest, sprinkle with chilli flakes and dollop on a couple of spoonfuls of the pesto.

3 / Add two or three stems of broccoli to the side, drizzle with a little olive oil and lift the edges of the foil up to wrap into a loose parcel, leaving some space for the ingredients to steam, and making sure that it is well sealed.

4 / Bake in the oven for 15–20 minutes. Carefully unravel one of the parcels to check the fattest part of the salmon; if it is pale pink all the way through it is done. If not, return to the oven for a further 5 minutes and check again.

An awesome dish to make if you have friends coming over, enchiladas win every time. If you can't get your hands on the chipotles you can always use a normal red chilli, and if you're after a veggie version swap the chicken for some sweet potato, courgette and mushrooms. A margarita wouldn't go amiss either!

Chicken enchiladas

||||||||||||||||||||||||||||||||||||||||||||||||||||||||||||||||||||||||||||||||||||||||||||||||

// SERVES 4 //

2 tbsp oil

3 boneless chicken breasts, cut into 2cm chunks

1 red onion, finely chopped

2 garlic cloves

1 tsp ground cumin

2 tsp ground coriander

pinch cayenne pepper

1 tsp paprika

1–2 tinned chipotles in adobo, chopped

1 x 400g tin tomatoes

1 tbsp tomato purée

150ml stock or water

juice of ½ lime

8 corn tortillas

1 red pepper, deseeded and thinly sliced

65g grated mozzarella, plus extra to sprinkle

sea salt and freshly ground black pepper

TO SERVE
soured cream

guacamole or avocado slices

1 / Preheat the oven to 190°C/Gas 5.

2 / Heat half the oil in a large pan and brown the chicken over medium-high heat all over. Remove from the pan and set aside.

3 / Add the remaining oil and fry the onions for 10 minutes, until translucent and soft. Stir in the garlic for 2 minutes, then add the spices and cook for another minute. Stir in the chipotles, tomatoes, tomato purée and stock and simmer, uncovered, for 15–20 minutes until slightly reduced. Add the lime juice and season well to taste.

4 / Grease a baking dish with a little oil. Take one tortilla and add some of the chicken pieces, a few slices of pepper and a bit of cheese. Roll firmly and place, seam side down, in the dish. Repeat with the remaining tortillas and filling.

5 / Pour the tomato sauce over the top and sprinkle with extra grated cheese.

6 / Bake for 35–40 minutes, until the cheese is bubbling and nicely melted. Serve with soured cream and guacamole or slices of avocado.

This is such a versatile dish – great with pasta or rice, you can also swap the Parmesan for some feta, as we've done here, or the lamb for turkey. Our favourite way to serve this is with polenta wedges, using the ready-made packs that you can get in supermarkets; simply slice and fry or bake until golden.

Spicy lamb meatballs

|||||||||||||||||||||||||||||||||||||||||||||||||||||||||||||||||||||||||||||||||||||||||||||||||||||||||||||

// SERVES 4 //

2 tbsp olive oil, plus extra to drizzle
1 small onion, thinly sliced
4 garlic cloves, sliced
400g tinned tomatoes
1 tbsp tomato purée
½ small red chilli, deseeded
  and finely sliced
sprig rosemary, leaves picked
  and thinly chopped
120ml chicken stock
finely grated Parmesan, to garnish
salad leaves, to serve (optional)

MEATBALLS
300g minced lamb
250g pork sausage meat,
  from about 3 sausages
1½ tsp fennel seeds
1 egg, beaten
pinch dried chilli flakes
sea salt and freshly ground black
  pepper

1 / Preheat the oven to 220°C/Gas 7.

2 / Make the sauce by heating the oil in a pan over medium-high heat. Add the onion and cook for 7–10 minutes, until softened. Add the garlic and cook for 1 minute, until slightly golden, then tip in the tomatoes. Stir in the tomato purée, chilli, rosemary and chicken stock, then bring to the boil. Reduce the heat and simmer for 15–20 minutes.

3 / To make the meatballs, line a baking tray with baking parchment. In a large bowl, combine all the ingredients and shape the mixture into golfball-sized meatballs. Arrange on the tray and drizzle with a little oil. (If you want to check the seasoning of the meat, before rolling them into balls, fry up a small amount in a pan and adjust the seasoning to taste.)

4 / Bake the meatballs in the oven for 20–25 minutes, until browned.

5 / Topple the meatballs into the sauce, and simmer over low heat for 5 minutes. Serve the meatballs with a few gratings of Parmesan together with the tomato sauce and some salad on the side. Alternatively serve the tomato sauce on the side as more of a dip. This is also great served with spaghetti.

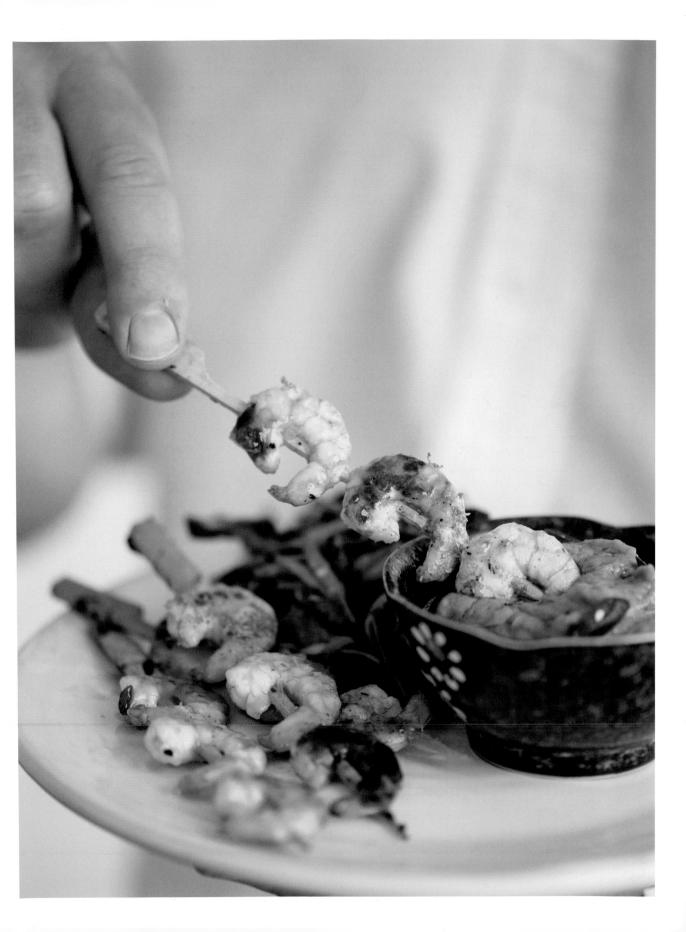

The colours of this are amazing and so uplifting when made on a chilly autumn evening; this is stuffed squash as it should be. You can swap the rice for quinoa or even some fried lamb mince, but we have to say the straight-up veggie version is our favourite.

Stuffed butternut squash

|||||||||||||||||||||||||||||||||||||||||||||||||||||||||||||||||||||||||||||||||||||||||||||||||||||

// SERVES 2 //

1 medium butternut squash
1 tbsp olive oil, plus extra
  for rubbing
100g basmati and wild rice
1 tsp sumac
1 garlic clove, crushed
6 spring onions
zest of ½ lemon
½ small bunch (25g) flat-leaf parsley,
  chopped
100g feta cheese
2–3 tbsp pomegranate seeds
sea salt and freshly ground black
  pepper
green salad, to serve

1 / Preheat the oven to 190°C/Gas 5.

2 / Slice the butternut in half and rub oil and salt and pepper all over it. Place the two halves in a baking tray, cut side down, and roast in the oven for 30 minutes.

3 / Meanwhile, put the rice in a saucepan and cover with twice the volume of water. Put the lid on the pan and cook over medium heat for 20 minutes, until the rice is tender and the water has all been absorbed. Set aside.

4 / Once the butternut has been cooking for 30 minutes, remove from the oven and turn the halves over. Sprinkle half the sumac over each half and return to the oven for another 15 minutes, or until the flesh has cooked through. Check by inserting a knife into the thickest part of the squash; if there is still resistance, return to the oven until it is cooked throughout.

5 / Heat the tablespoon of olive oil in a frying pan and cook the garlic and spring onions gently for a few minutes. Add the rice, lemon zest and most of the parsley and stir everything together. Crumble in about half of the feta and season well with salt and pepper.

6 / Remove the squash from the oven again and fill the holes with the rice stuffing. Crumble the remaining feta over the top of the rice and return to the oven for about 10 minutes, until the feta has melted.

7 / Sprinkle the squash with the reserved parsley and pomegranate seeds and serve with a green salad.

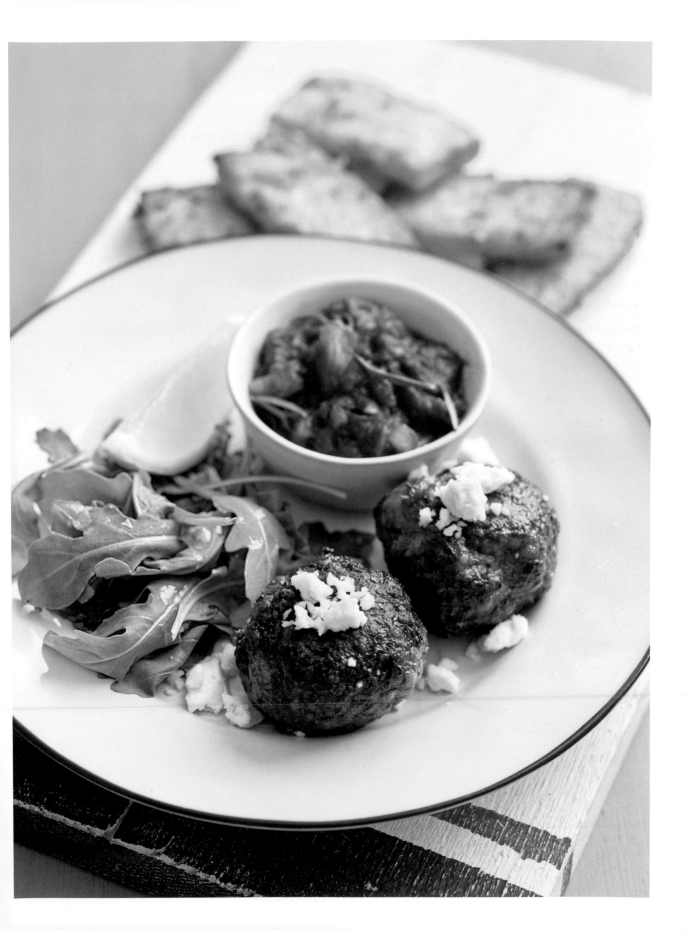

This is our take on a takeaway classic: fresher, lighter and less sugary than what often turns up in a plastic tray. Add some steamed rice if you're in need of a little more sustenance, or alternatively serve as a help-yourself starter if you're having people over. If you have any leftover satay sauce thin it down with a little more lime juice and use like a dressing for a big green salad.

Satay prawn dippers

|||||||||||||||||||||||||||||||||||||||||||||||||||||||||||||||||||||||||||||||||||||||||||||||||

// MAKES 6 SKEWERS //

1 tbsp olive oil
juice of 1 lime
1½ tbsp fish sauce
1 red chilli, deseeded
  and finely chopped
thumb-sized piece ginger,
  finely chopped
3 garlic cloves, finely chopped
½ tsp ground turmeric
24 raw tiger prawns, peeled
2 tsp honey

SATAY SAUCE
2 tbsp coconut or peanut oil
2 shallots or ½ small onion,
  finely chopped
1 garlic clove, finely chopped
1cm piece ginger, finely chopped
2 tbsp soy sauce
2 heaped tbsp crunchy peanut butter
200ml coconut cream
juice of ½ lime

QUICK ASIAN SLAW
2 tbsp soy sauce
juice of ½ lime
1 tbsp sesame oil
½ head red cabbage, shredded
2 medium carrots, grated
handful fresh coriander, leaves
  picked and chopped
1 tbsp sesame seeds

1 / Whisk the olive oil, lime juice and fish sauce with the chilli, ginger, garlic and turmeric. Add the prawns and honey and stir well. Cover with clingfilm and marinate for 30 minutes.

2 / Meanwhile, make the satay sauce. Heat the oil in a pan and fry the shallots or onion, garlic and ginger until softened. Add the soy sauce, peanut butter and coconut cream. Stir in the lime juice and soy sauce, adding more, if needed, to taste.

3 / Assemble the quick Asian slaw. Whisk together the soy sauce, lime juice and sesame oil in a large bowl. Add the red cabbage, carrots, coriander and sesame seeds and toss to coat with the dressing; set aside.

4 / To cook the prawns, heat a griddle pan over high heat until very hot. Thread 4 prawns onto each skewer and cook for 3 minutes per side, or until the prawns are pink and opaque. Serve with the Asian slaw and the satay sauce for dipping.

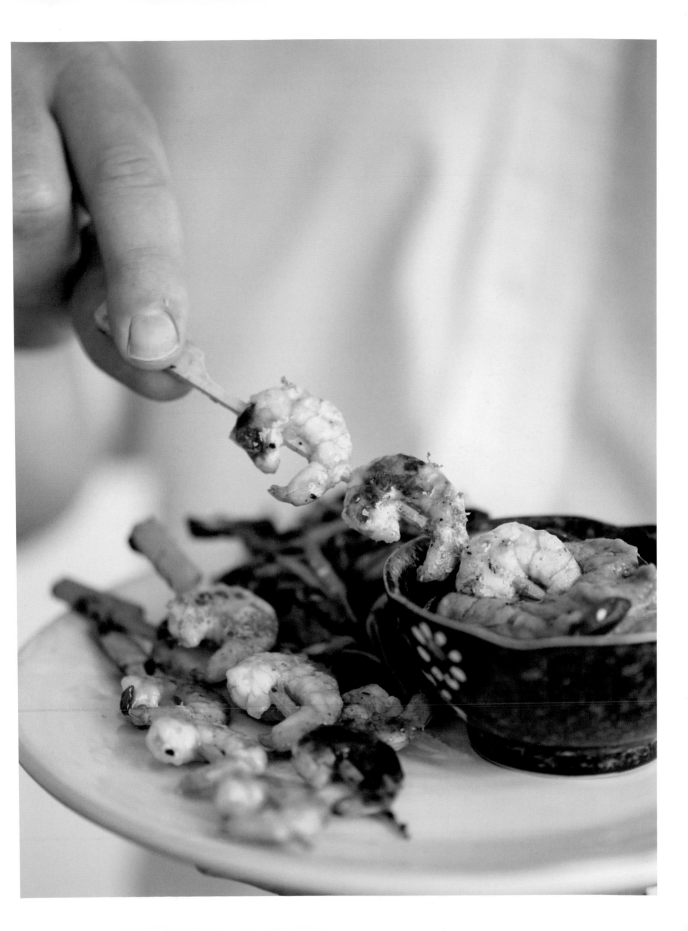

The colours of this are amazing and so uplifting when made on a chilly autumn evening; this is stuffed squash as it should be. You can swap the rice for quinoa or even some fried lamb mince, but we have to say the straight-up veggie version is our favourite.

Stuffed butternut squash

||||||||||||||||||||||||||||||||||||||||||||||||||||||||||||||||||||||||||||||||||||||||||||||||||||||||

// SERVES 2 //

1 medium butternut squash
1 tbsp olive oil, plus extra
  for rubbing
100g basmati and wild rice
1 tsp sumac
1 garlic clove, crushed
6 spring onions
zest of ½ lemon
½ small bunch (25g) flat-leaf parsley,
  chopped
100g feta cheese
2–3 tbsp pomegranate seeds
sea salt and freshly ground black
  pepper
green salad, to serve

1 / Preheat the oven to 190°C/Gas 5.

2 / Slice the butternut in half and rub oil and salt and pepper all over it. Place the two halves in a baking tray, cut side down, and roast in the oven for 30 minutes.

3 / Meanwhile, put the rice in a saucepan and cover with twice the volume of water. Put the lid on the pan and cook over medium heat for 20 minutes, until the rice is tender and the water has all been absorbed. Set aside.

4 / Once the butternut has been cooking for 30 minutes, remove from the oven and turn the halves over. Sprinkle half the sumac over each half and return to the oven for another 15 minutes, or until the flesh has cooked through. Check by inserting a knife into the thickest part of the squash; if there is still resistance, return to the oven until it is cooked throughout.

5 / Heat the tablespoon of olive oil in a frying pan and cook the garlic and spring onions gently for a few minutes. Add the rice, lemon zest and most of the parsley and stir everything together. Crumble in about half of the feta and season well with salt and pepper.

6 / Remove the squash from the oven again and fill the holes with the rice stuffing. Crumble the remaining feta over the top of the rice and return to the oven for about 10 minutes, until the feta has melted.

7 / Sprinkle the squash with the reserved parsley and pomegranate seeds and serve with a green salad.

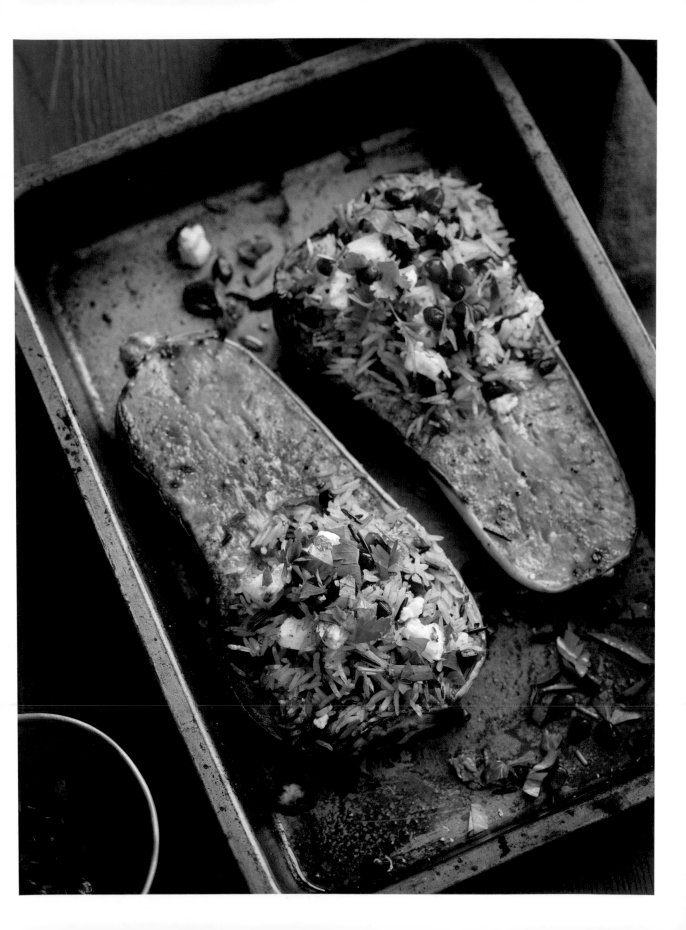

We are not claiming this as an authentic Italian risotto, but it is certainly delicious. The quinoa gives a great texture and extra nutrition boost, while mixing it with the rice keeps the dish affordable. Easily doubled, swap the chicken stock for veggie and use a vegetarian Parmesan if you want to make it meat-free.

Quinoa & mushroom 'risotto'

// SERVES 2 //

25g dried porcini mushrooms
1 tbsp plus 2 tsp coconut oil
3 garlic cloves, finely chopped
150g chestnut mushrooms
   (or mixed), sliced
1 onion, finely chopped
70g quinoa
80g risotto rice
1 glass white wine
600–750ml hot chicken stock
zest of ½ lemon
25g Parmesan, grated
sea salt and freshly ground
   black pepper
handful flat-leaf parsley leaves,
   to serve

1 / Soak the dried mushrooms in 3 tablespoons of boiling water for 10 minutes.

2 / Heat 1 teaspoon of oil in a large frying pan and add half the garlic. Squeeze the mushrooms dry, reserving the liquid in the bowl, and add these to the pan. Let the mushrooms cook for 3–4 minutes, then add the reserved mushroom-soaking liquid. Bubble on high for 2–3 minutes, to reduce slightly, then put the mix into a bowl.

3 / Add another teaspoon of oil to the pan and fry the sliced mushrooms over high heat, to brown them. Season with salt and pepper and remove to the bowl with the porcini mushrooms. Set aside

4 / Heat the remaining oil in the same pan over medium heat. Add the onion and remaining garlic, and cook for 10–15 minutes, until soft and translucent. Add the quinoa and rice, stirring to coat in the oil.

5 / Turn up the heat to medium-high and pour in the wine. Let it bubble away for a few minutes, until the grains absorb the wine. Add one ladleful of the hot stock and stir through, letting the rice and quinoa absorb the liquid almost completely, before adding another ladle of stock. Continue to do this for 20–30 minutes, until the rice and quinoa are just tender to bite.

6 / Next, stir in the mushrooms along with the juices in the bowl and heat through for 5 minutes. Finally, add the lemon zest, season to taste and stir through the Parmesan. Garnish with parsley and serve.

We are big fans of any dish that makes the most of inexpensive cuts of meat; braising beef takes longer to cook but it is definitely worth it, and actually sometimes taking your time over a slow-cook one-pot is a lot more enjoyable (not to mention relaxing) than manically chucking things in a frying pan on a 30-second timer. This freezes really well too, so double up and you'll be smug in the knowledge that you've got a hearty meal ready for you when you need it.

Beef tagine

// SERVES 4 //

rapeseed or olive oil, for frying
1 large onion, finely chopped
2 garlic cloves, finely chopped
500g braising beef, diced into chunky
   pieces
700g passata
1 beef jelly stock cube dissolved
   in 300ml hot water
3 tbsp harissa paste
1 x 400g tin chickpeas, rinsed
   and drained
200g stoned prunes, chopped
   in half
sea salt and freshly ground
   black pepper
couscous, to serve
chopped parsley, to sprinkle

1 / Heat a little oil in a large casserole dish and fry the onion and garlic for 6–7 minutes over low–medium heat, until the onions are softened and translucent.

2 / Add the beef and fry for another 2–3 minutes until the beef is browned all over, then add the passata and beef stock. Stir through the harissa and bring the mixture to the boil. Reduce the heat to low and pop a lid on the pan. Cook for 1½ hours, until the meat is really tender, stirring from time to time.

3 / Remove the lid and cook for a further 30 minutes to reduce and thicken the liquid. Add the chickpeas and prunes to the mixture and cook for a further 5–10 minutes to warm them through; you should now have a really deep-brown, rich sauce.

4 / Season really well with salt and pepper and serve with couscous and a little chopped parsley sprinkled over the top.

Inside-out, outside-in – whichever way you look at it these burgers are the bomb. Feel free to experiment with the filling – blue cheese and a little chopped bacon, red onion jam and goat's cheese… endless opportunities! You can also make little mini ones and pretend you're a giant :-)

The Inside-out burger

||||||||||||||||||||||||||||||||||||||||||||||||||||||||||||||||||||||||||||||||||||||||||

// SERVES 2 //

300g minced beef
handful breadcrumbs
2 tsp chopped thyme
2 dashes Worcestershire sauce
150g spinach leaves
4 tbsp coarsely grated mozzarella
  cheese
2–3 jarred roasted red peppers, finely
  sliced
sea salt and freshly ground
  black pepper
oil, for frying

TO SERVE
2 brioche burger buns or 4 mini buns
gherkins, sliced
1 avocado, de-stoned and sliced
tomato sauce and/or mustard sauce

1 / In a large bowl, combine the mince, breadcrumbs, thyme and Worcestershire sauce and season with salt and pepper. Divide the mixture into 4 large balls and place on a tray lined with parchment paper. Chill in the fridge for 30 minutes.

2 / Meanwhile, blanch the spinach in a pan of boiling water for 1 minute. Drain and rinse under cold running water. When cool, use your hands to squeeze as much moisture out of the spinach as possible. You won't be left with much spinach but you don't need much for the burgers!

3 / Remove the burgers from the fridge and flatten each one out into a 1cm patty, roughly. Put about half of the mozzarella on one patty, followed by a few pieces of red pepper and a little bit of spinach. Take another patty and place on top to sandwich the two together, then squeeze the edges to seal and enclose the fillings. Repeat with the remaining patties.

4 / Heat the oil in a frying pan over medium–high heat. Add the burgers. You may want to do this one at a time depending on how large your pan is. Fry for 6–8 minutes on each side over medium heat or until cooked to your preference.

5 / Take off the heat and drain on kitchen paper.

6 / As these are cooking, grill your buns on the cut sides. Serve the burgers on a toasted bun half and top with gherkins, avocado slices and tomato sauce or whichever condiments you like.

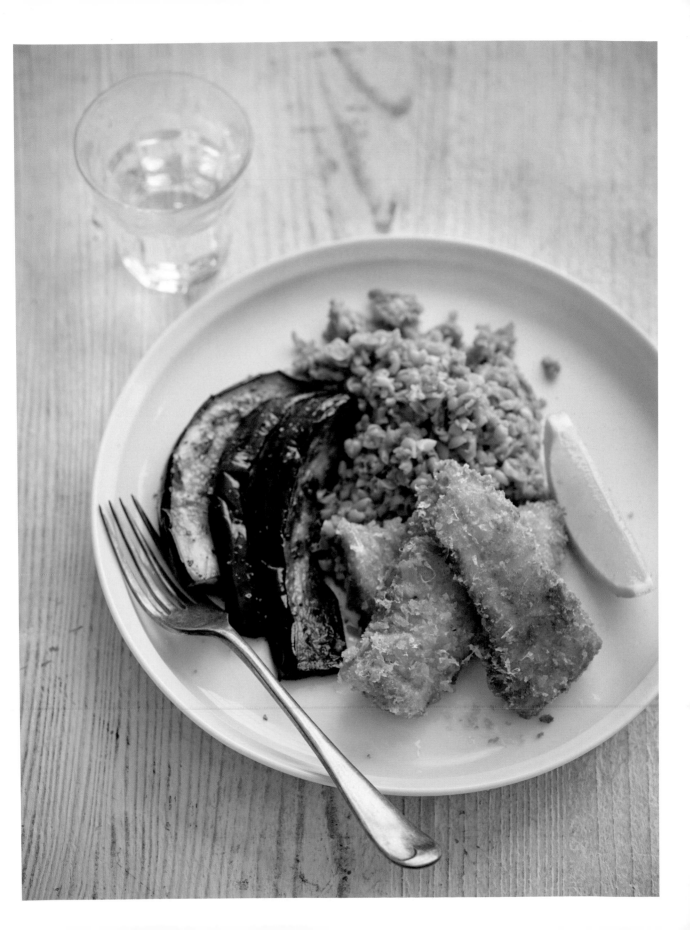

Everyone needs a good roast recipe up their sleeve (well maybe 'needs' is a little strong, but you see where we're going with this) and here is our favourite version, courtesy of our pal Alex, AKA @thefoodgrinder

The creamy dauphinoise puts it a little more on the indulgent side, but hey, it's a roast – who cooks a roast every day? So tuck in and enjoy!

The Food Grinder Roast with sweet potato dauphinoise

||||||||||||||||||||||||||||||||||||||||||||||||||||||||||||||||||||||||||||||||||||||||||

// SERVES 6 //

1 large whole chicken, the best quality you can afford
1 small bunch fresh rosemary
1 small bunch fresh thyme
60g butter
1 lemon, zested
½ red onion, halved again
1 whole garlic bulb, halved widthwise
sea salt and freshly ground black pepper

DAUPHINOISE
1kg sweet potatoes
750ml double cream

KALE SALAD
1 x 180g bag kale
3 tbsp extra virgin olive oil
2 tbsp lemon juice
½ red chilli, very finely diced
sea salt and freshly ground black pepper

1 / Preheat the oven to 200°C/Gas 6. Weigh the bird and calculate the roasting time, giving it 20 minutes for every 500g, plus an extra 20 minutes.

2 / Strip half of the rosemary and thyme leaves from their stalks and chop very finely; leave aside a spoonful of herbs for the dauphinoise. Mix the chopped herbs with the butter, lemon zest and a bit of seasoning. Carefully lift up the skin of the chicken, separating it from the meat, and spread the butter all over the top of the bird under the skin.

3 / Slice the zested lemon in half and place it in the cavity of the chicken, along with the onion, garlic bulb and the rest of the herbs. Roast for the calculated cooking time, covering the bird with a piece of foil if it begins to start looking a bit brown on top.

4 / While the chicken is roasting, prepare the dauphinoise. Slice the potatoes into 2–3mm slices – a mandoline is easiest for this. Lay them in a buttered rectangular baking dish.

continued....

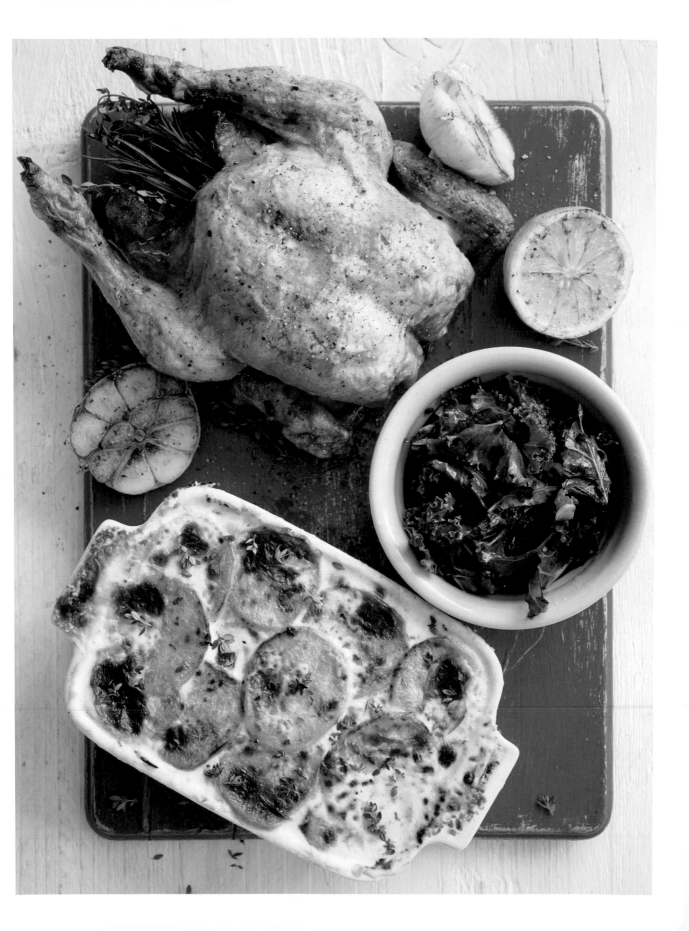

5 / Put the cream along with the rosemary and thyme in a saucepan and heat to just simmering. Season really well with salt and pepper and pour over the potato slices in the baking dish. Put the dauphinoise in the oven with the chicken for the last hour of cooking.

6 / While the chicken and dauphinoise are cooking, prepare the kale salad. Put the kale in a bowl and drizzle over the oil and lemon juice. Using your hands, massage the dressing into the kale. Keep going for a good 5–10 minutes as the massaging will tenderise the kale. Add the chopped chilli and season well with salt and pepper.

7 / Remove the chicken from the oven and check that the juices run clear when pierced in the thickest place with a knife. Check that the dauphinoise is cooked by inserting a knife into the centre – if it goes in easily without any resistance, it is done. Serve the chicken with the dauphinoise and kale salad.

The colours in this when sliced are awesome and look pretty fancy too. You'll need to expend a little more effort than if you were just whacking a steak in a pan, but the extra flavours you get are absolutely worth it. A dish to impress with.

Stuffed rolled steak with sweet potato wedges

||||||||||||||||||||||||||||||||||||||||||||||||||||||||||||||||||||||||||||||||||||||||||||||||

// SERVES 4 //

700g flank or bavette steak,
 in one long piece
6 slices prosciutto
125g ball mozzarella, sliced thinly
handful basil leaves
1 tbsp olive oil
sea salt and freshly ground black
 pepper
1 quantity Sweet Potato Wedges
 (see page 104), to serve

JAMES'S TIP

This goes great with a simple rocket and tomato salad; simply toss some rocket with sliced tomatoes, add a little lemon juice and a drizzle of olive oil.

1 / Preheat the oven to 190°C/Gas 5.

2 / Put the steak between 2 sheets of clingfilm and bash with a rolling pin to thin it to 1cm thick and to tenderise it. Remove the top layer of clingfilm and season well with salt and pepper.

3 / Lay the prosciutto slices over the entire surface of the steak. On top of that, lay the mozzarella slices, leaving a couple of inches clear at one end, followed by the basil leaves. Turn the steak so it's widthways on to you and the space without the cheese is at the far end. Start rolling up the steak from the nearest end, firmly but not too tightly, as you don't want the cheese to be squeezed out. Once you have a roll, tie it up with pieces of string at 4cm intervals, again not pulling it too tight, and making sure the knots in the string are on the underside of the roll, where the seam is.

4 / Heat the oil in a frying pan with an ovenproof handle until very hot. Sear the steak roll for about 5 minutes, turning regularly, until it is browned all over. Transfer the pan to the oven and roast for about 35 minutes if you'd like it quite pink in the middle. Cook for another 5–10 minutes if you'd like it more well done. Remove the steak from the hot pan and place on a chopping board, cover with a sheet of foil, and leave to rest for about 10 minutes before carving.

5 / Serve slices of the steak roll with the sweet potato wedges.

When we say any fish, we mean any fish; if its got fins, it will probably work. The combination of roasted fennel, lemon, garlic and new potatoes is such a good one it goes with everything from salmon to sea bass. This is definitely a recipe where it's worth experimenting with the more sustainable (and often cheaper) types of fish such as coley and pollock.

Any-fish traybake

||||||||||||||||||||||||||||||||||||||||||||||||||||||||||||||||||||||||||||||||||||||||||

// SERVES 2 //

1 red pepper
1 whole garlic head
1 red onion
½ lemon, cut into wedges
1 fennel bulb, cut into 6 wedges
1 tsp pink peppercorns
10 small new potatoes, sliced
1 tsp fennel seeds
extra virgin olive oil, to drizzle
250g spinach leaves
2 thick white fish fillets,
  such as brill or sea bass
sea salt and freshly ground
  black pepper

1 / Preheat the oven to 200°C/Gas 6.

2 / Slice the pepper in half, remove the core and seeds and cut the pepper into 1.5cm thick slices. Throw into a roasting tin.

3 / Slice the garlic across the equator, not pole to pole, and throw that in to the tin with the pepper. Add the lemon wedges, fennel wedges, peppercorns, potatoes and fennel seeds. Drizzle with oil, season with salt and pepper and toss, using your hands, so everything is coated.

4 / Put in the oven for 35–40 minutes, until the fennel has softened and the garlic turned golden.

5 / Meanwhile, bring a pan of water to the boil and blanch the spinach for 30 seconds, drain and rinse under cold water. Squeeze out as much water as you can from the spinach to prevent the dish becoming watery.

6 / Take the veggies out of the oven and arrange the fish fillets over the top. Scatter with the spinach, season with salt and pepper, and return to the oven for 12–15 minutes, or until the fish is opaque and cooked through. Serve immediately with a drizzle of extra virgin olive oil.

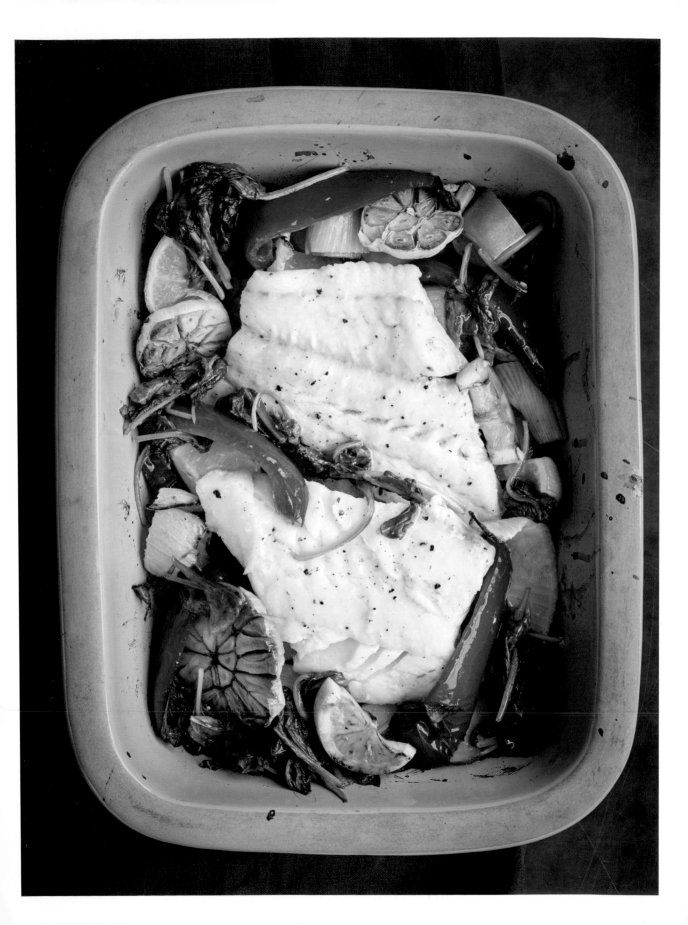

Any dish that involves halloumi is a winner in our books, and this one is no exception. Packed full of veg, this is as healthy as it is hearty. Adding the toasted coconut and cashews gives a little unexpected twist, and adds a great warmth and depth to the dish.

Rainbow rice

||||||||||||||||||||||||||||||||||||||||||||||||||||||||||||||||||||||||||||||||||||||||||||||

// SERVES 2–3 //

1 tbsp coconut oil

½ red onion, finely chopped

1 garlic clove, finely diced

1 red and 1 green pepper,
  cored and finely chopped

1 courgette, finely diced

185g brown rice

5 rainbow chard leaves,
  roughly chopped

435ml chicken or vegetable stock

125g halloumi, cut into 2cm squares

handful of cashew nuts

handful of desiccated coconut

2 spring onions, thinly sliced

extra virgin olive oil, to serve

sea salt and freshly ground
  black pepper

1 / Heat the oil in a flameproof casserole pan. Fry the onion and garlic for 10 minutes, until soft. Add the peppers and courgette and cook for 5–10 minutes. Stir in the rice and chard, and let it cook for just a minute. Then pour over the stock. Season with salt and pepper.

2 / Cut a circle of baking parchment the size of the pan and sit it on top of the surface of the rice. Put the lid on top and cook over very low heat for 20–30 minutes, or until the rice has absorbed most of the liquid and is tender to bite. Take off the heat and leave to sit for 10 minutes.

3 / Meanwhile, heat a frying pan with a dash of oil. Add the halloumi and fry until golden on both sides. Remove to drain on kitchen paper. Wipe round the pan with a little more kitchen roll, then tip in the cashews and coconut. Toss them around the pan to lightly toast.

4 / Take the lid off the pan and fold through the halloumi, coconut, spring onions and cashews. Drizzle with a little olive oil and serve at room temperature.

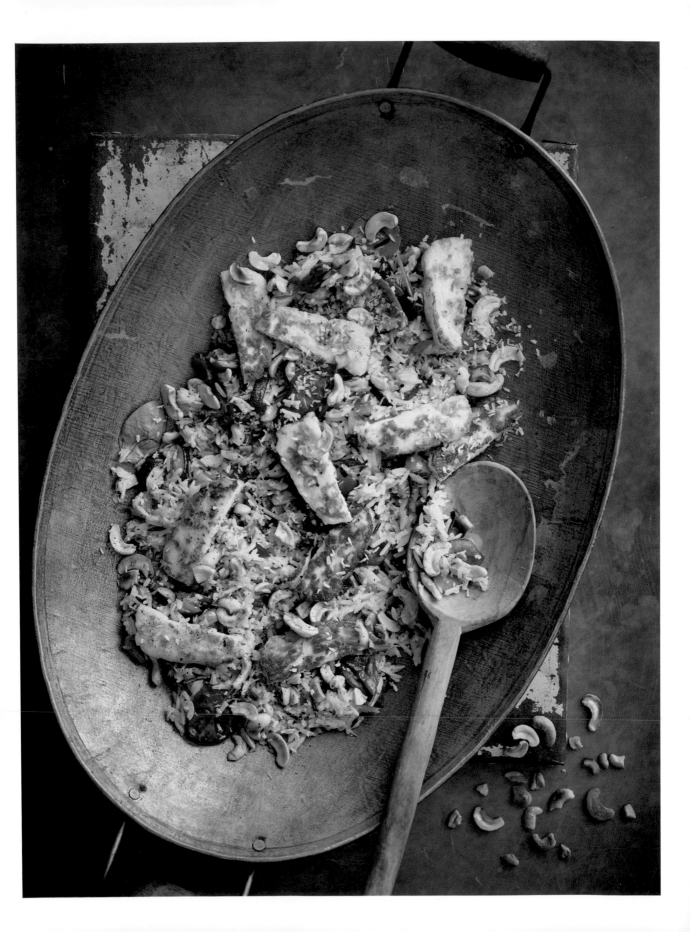

Snacks
& on the go

||||||||||||||||||||||||||||||||||||||||||||

Just like a good roast, it's worth having a hummus recipe in your repertoire. Here you've got a classic version and three variations – the beetroot is our favourite if only for the colour it goes. Serve with crudités, pitta or wholemeal tortilla chips (see page 46).

Hummus 4 ways

// SERVES 4–6 //

1 × 400g tin chickpeas, rinsed and drained
1 plump garlic clove, peeled and roughly chopped
juice of 1½ lemons
4 tbsp olive oil
2 tbsp tahini
2 tbsp natural yoghurt
1 tsp sea salt
smoked paprika, to sprinkle
extra virgin olive oil, to drizzle

CLASSIC

1 / Put the chickpeas in a food processor and process to a stiff paste. Add the garlic, lemon juice, olive oil, tahini, yoghurt and salt. Blitz again, then slowly drizzle in 1–2 tablespoons ice-cold water, mixing for another 3 minutes, until you have a smooth paste and to your desired consistency. Adjust the seasoning, to taste.

2 / Transfer to a bowl and let the hummus sit in the fridge for 30 minutes, to allow the garlic to mellow.

BEETROOT AND FETA

Add 3 tinned or vacuum-packed beetroots, drained. Omit the paprika and serve with crumbled feta and a few nigella seeds over the top.

CANNELLI BEANS, PEAS AND MINT

Replace the chickpeas with cannellini beans. Add a handful of fresh and cooked peas and plenty of mint, and omit the paprika.

ROASTED RED PEPPER

Add 1–2 roasted and peeled red peppers from a jar.

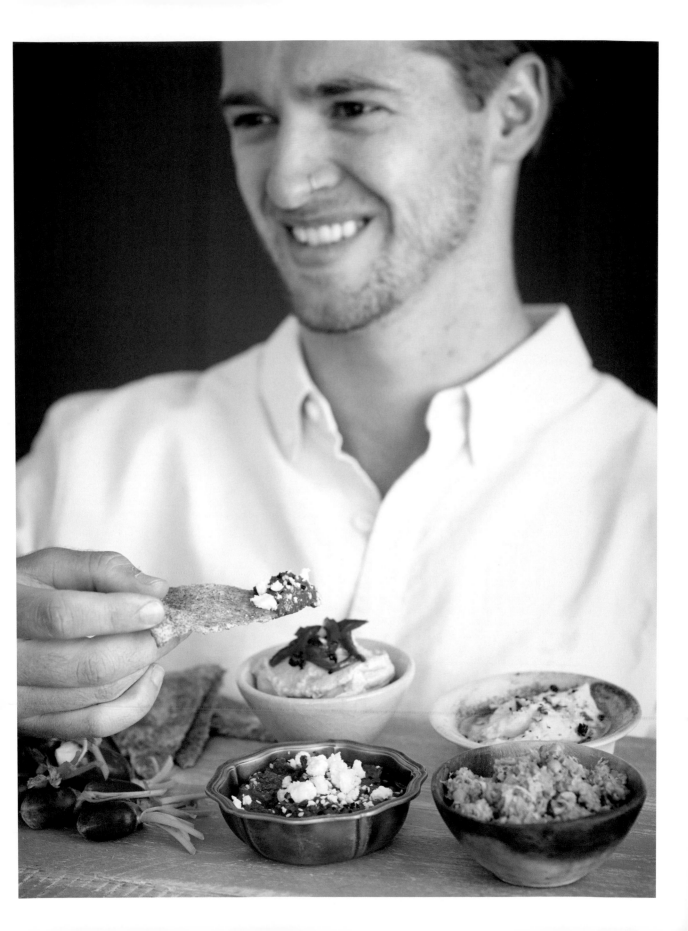

Much lighter than your average muffin, these gluten-free mini frittatas make a great snack and are equally good for breakfast. Courgette and feta is our favourite filling, but peas, cheddar, a little roast sweet potato or mushrooms work well too.

Courgette & feta frittata muffins

// MAKES 8 //

butter or oil, for greasing
120g grated courgette
  (about 1 small courgette)
6 large eggs
small handful mint leaves,
  finely chopped
100g feta cheese, diced into
  5mm cubes
sea salt and freshly ground
  black pepper

1 / Preheat the oven to 180°C/Gas 4 and grease really well 8 holes of a non-stick muffin tin.

2 / Sandwich the grated courgette between several sheets of kitchen paper and press down on the paper to squeeze out as much water as you can.

3 / Whisk the eggs, then stir in the grated courgette, chopped mint and most of the feta cubes. Season the mixture really well with black pepper and a little salt, remembering that the cheese is quite salty.

4 / Divide the mixture evenly between the holes of the muffin tin and sprinkle the remaining feta over the top of the mixture. Bake for about 18 minutes, or until the frittatas are risen, golden and cooked through. Remove from the tin while still warm or they may stick.

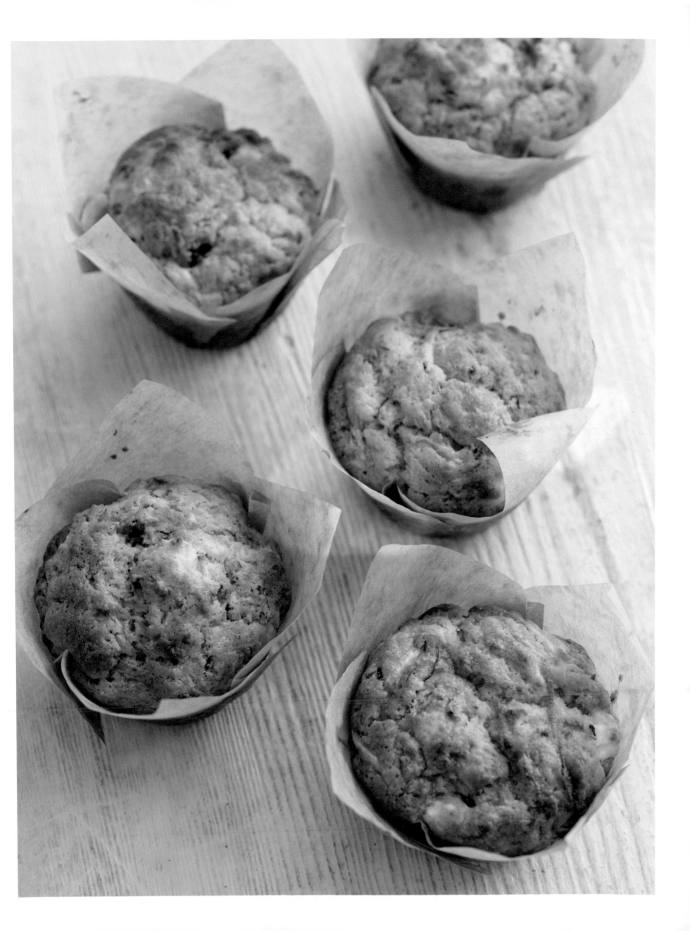

These taste even better than they look. And there's something distinctly chocolate-bar-with-nuts-and-caramel about the bars...

Protein truffles

||||||||||||||||||||||||||||||||||||||||||||||||||||||||||||||||||||||||||||||||||||||||||||||||||||||

// MAKES APPROX. 12 //

100g dark chocolate
100g ground almonds
1 tbsp maple syrup
1 tbsp whey protein (chocolate or
vanilla flavour work well)

TOPPINGS
Chopped nuts (hazelnuts work well)
Desiccated coconut

1 / Get yourself a big heatproof bowl and place over a pan of simmering water. Break the chocolate over it and leave to melt (don't stir the chocolate while it's melting). Take off the heat, stir in the almonds, maple syrup and whey protein to combine. Stick the bowl in the fridge for an hour or so.

2 / Remove from the fridge and use your hands to scoop little balls of the mixture - which should have hardened slightly – and roll in a topping of your choice. We find that scattering the toppings on a large plate works well. Stick back in the fridge for another hour to set, then try not to eat them all at once!

PB-cookie-dough bars

||||||||||||||||||||||||||||||||||||||||||||||||||||||||||||||||||||||||||||||||||||||||||||||||||||||

MAKES APPROX. 16 BARS

3 tbsp peanut butter
(smooth or crunchy)
1 tsp vanilla essence or extract
80g dark-chocolate chips
100g ground almonds
1 tbsp honey or maple syrup
1 tbsp whey protein
(chocolate or vanilla work well)
melted chocolate for drizzling
(optional)

1 / Melt the peanut butter with the vanilla, either in the microwave or in a heatproof bowl set over simmering water. Stir in the ground almonds and honey, and mix well to combine. Leave to cool a little then mix in the whey protein and dark-chocolate chips till you have a big ball of cookie-dough-like consistency. Flatten the ball into a tray lined with baking parchment, so that it is evenly spread out and roughly 2cm thick. Chill in the fridge for a couple of hours.

2 / To up the chocolate ante, melt a little dark chocolate and drizzle over the top before putting in the fridge to chill. Looks pretty too.

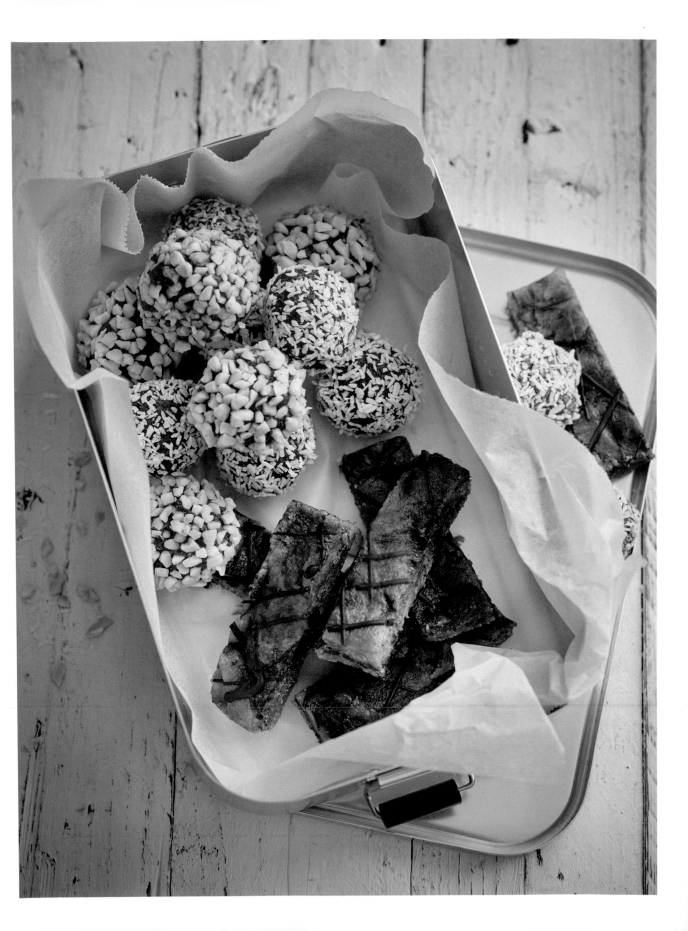

These are light, fluffy and a world away from the dry pretenders you get in shops. The grated apple adds a natural sweetness, but if you're after a little more sweet for your buck, check out Tom's tip below.

Carrot & walnut muffins

|||||||||||||||||||||||||||||||||||||||||||||||||||||||||||||||||||||||||||||||||||||||||||

// MAKES 12 //

300g white spelt flour

2 tsp ground cinnamon

2 tsp baking powder

pinch table salt

100g mild, odourless coconut oil

150ml maple syrup, plus extra
to drizzle (optional – see below)

2 large eggs, beaten

125g grated carrot (about 1 large
carrot, peeled)

125g grated apple (about 1 apple,
peeled)

100g walnuts, roughly chopped

1 / Preheat the oven to 190°C/Gas 5 and line a 12-hole muffin tin with paper cases (the parchment tulip ones are good for these).

2 / Combine all the dry ingredients in a large mixing bowl.

3 / Melt the coconut oil in a pan over gentle heat. Remove from the heat and mix in the maple syrup.

4 / Make a well in the centre of the dry ingredients and pour in the oil and syrup mixture, beaten eggs, grated carrot and apple, and two-thirds of the walnuts. Mix together with a large spoon until just incorporated – be careful not to overmix or the mixture may be tough.

5 / Spoon the mixture evenly between the muffin cases and sprinkle the remaining walnuts over the tops. Bake in the oven for 22 minutes, until cooked through and golden on top.

TOM 'S TIP

These are sweet, but not as tooth-achingly sweet as the coffee-shop muffins we have got used to. If you want them a little sweeter, just drizzle a bit more maple syrup over each muffin once they come out of the oven and are still warm.

The sweet stuff

||||||||||||||||||||||||||||||||||||||||||||||||||||||||

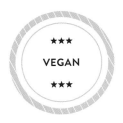

This is pretty much instant ice cream – no churners needed. Go for bananas that are little on the old side, as they will have a more intense natural sweetness.

Banana & chocolate (n)ice cream

// SERVES 2 //

2 bananas, peeled, sliced and frozen

1 tbsp raw cacao powder or 3 tbsp Nutella

2 tsp maple syrup or honey, or 1 date, chopped

½ tsp vanilla extract

pinch sea salt flakes

1 / Put the bananas in a food processor and blend until smooth, scraping down the sides occasionally. Add the cacao powder, maple, syrup, vanilla and salt and blend again to combine. Serve and enjoy.

2 / This can be made in advance and stored in the freezer for up to a day.

VARIATIONS

Try grating over fresh coconut or topping with chopped pistachio nuts or cashews. A small pinch of ground cardamom will also add a lovely spice dimension.

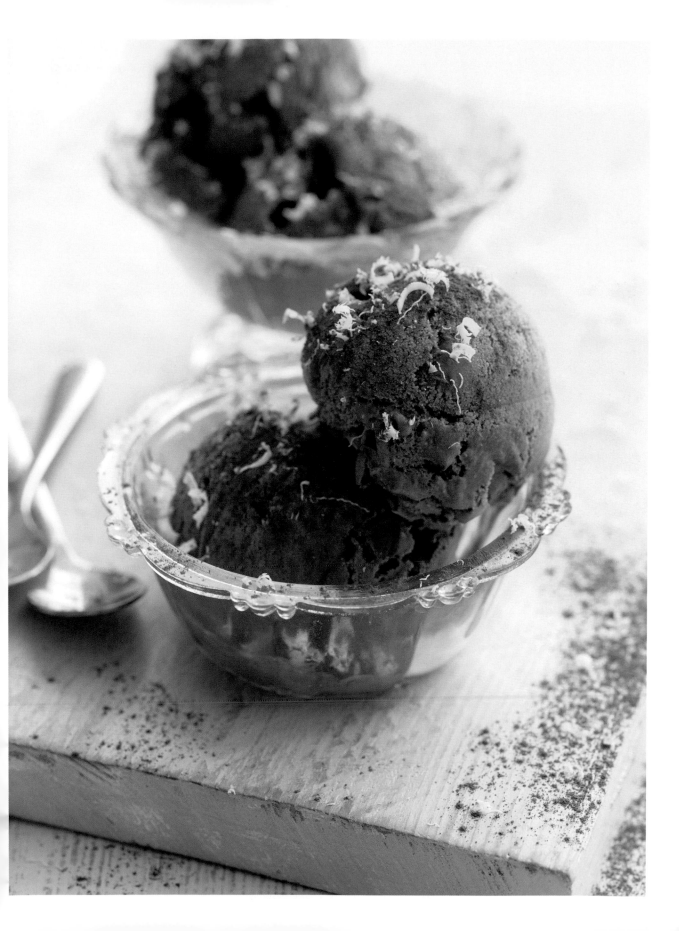

What the (n)ice cream said – the riper the banana the better. If you don't have much of a sweet tooth feel free to leave out the coconut sugar; on the other hand, if you are a more-the-merrier type when it comes to sweetness, chuck in a handful of dark chocolate chips. Once it's a day old this toasts brilliantly too.

Banana bread

||||||||||||||||||||||||||||||||||||||||||||||||||||||||||||||||||||||||||||||||||||||||

// MAKES 1 LOAF (8–10 SLICES) //

200g oats
1 tsp baking powder
½ tsp bicarbonate of soda
1 tsp ground cinnamon
pinch salt
2 large over-ripe bananas
1 tbsp crunchy peanut butter
40g coconut oil
40g coconut sugar
1 tbsp lemon juice
2 eggs, beaten

1 / Preheat the oven to 180°C/Gas 4 and grease and line a 450g loaf tin.

2 / Put the oats in a food processor and grind them down to a flour. Tip into a bowl and mix in the baking powder, bicarbonate of soda, cinnamon and salt. Set aside.

3 / Mash the bananas in a mixing bowl with a fork. Don't worry about getting them too smooth as the mixer will finish that off. Add the peanut butter, coconut oil, sugar and lemon juice and whisk with an electric hand whisk. Crack in the eggs and whisk again.

4 / Tip the dry ingredients into the banana mixture and fold in with a large spoon until well incorporated. Pour the mixture into the prepared loaf tin and spread evenly. Bake in the oven for 50 minutes–1 hour, or until a skewer inserted into the centre of the cake comes out clean. Check on it after 30 minutes, as you may need to cover the top of the loaf with a sheet of foil to stop the top going too dark. Allow the cake to cool in the tin for 10 minutes, then transfer to a wire rack to cool completely before slicing.

Recipes that involve vegetables and chocolate are no longer considered bonkers, for which we should all be thankful; from beetroot to courgette and aubergine, moist and dense veggies combined with good quality cocoa powder are a match made in heaven. Here the sweet potato flesh saves you having to add a tonne of butter and sugar to keep things sweet and fudgy.

Sweet potato brownies

// MAKES 12 //

3–4 medium sweet potatoes
  (to give you 300g mashed flesh)
150g crunchy sugar-free
  peanut butter
6 tbsp maple syrup
3 large eggs, beaten
60g cocoa powder
1 tsp baking powder

1 / Preheat the oven to 180°C/Gas 4 and grease and line a 20 x 25cm brownie tin.

2 / Put the sweet potatoes in the microwave and cook for about 8 minutes. Stick a knife in to check the potatoes are soft and cooked all the way through, and, if not, cook a little longer until they are. Scoop the flesh out of the potatoes and weigh out 300g (you can eat the remainder or use it in another dish).

3 / In a large mixing bowl, whisk together the sweet potato, peanut butter and maple syrup with an electric hand whisk until well combined, then whisk in the eggs.

4 / Sift the cocoa and baking powder into the bowl and fold everything together until well combined.

5 / Pour the batter into the prepared brownie tin and spread out evenly. Bake in the oven for 20 minutes, until risen and firm on top. Leave to cool for a few minutes in the tin, then transfer to a wire rack to cool completely.

6 / Cut into 12 slices to serve.

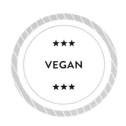

★★★

VEGAN

★★★

This is great served with a dollop of Greek yoghurt or crème fraiche, or to keep it vegan whip up a quick vanilla cream: whisk coconut cream with a teaspoon of vanilla essence and a grating of lemon zest.

Lemon polenta cake

// SERVES 8 //

90g fine polenta
55g ground almonds
120g plain flour
2½ tsp baking powder
pinch of salt
170g unrefined caster sugar
2 tbsp maple syrup
70ml rapeseed or grapeseed oil
250ml soy milk or almond milk
2 tsp cider vinegar
zest of 3 lemons
juice of 2 lemons

DRIZZLE
juice of 2 lemons
3 tbsp unrefined caster sugar

1 / Preheat the oven to 190°C/Gas 5. Grease and line a 20cm springform cake tin.

2 / Whisk together the polenta, ground almonds, flour and baking powder in a large bowl. Add the salt.

3 / In a separate bowl, combine the sugar, syrup, oil, milk, vinegar, lemon zest and juice, and stir well. Pour this mixture into the dry ingredients and stir until just combined.

4 / Transfer to the tin and bake for 35–45 minutes, until a skewer inserted into the middle of the cake comes out clean.

5 / About 5 minutes before the cake is due to come out of the oven, heat the lemon juice and caster sugar in a small pan and simmer until syrupy, about 5 minutes.

6 / Take the cake out of the oven and poke holes in the surface using a wooden skewer. Drizzle over the syrup, then leave the cake to cool in the tin for 10 minutes, before transferring to a wire rack to cool completely.

7 / Serve with yoghurt and grated lemon zest, if you like.

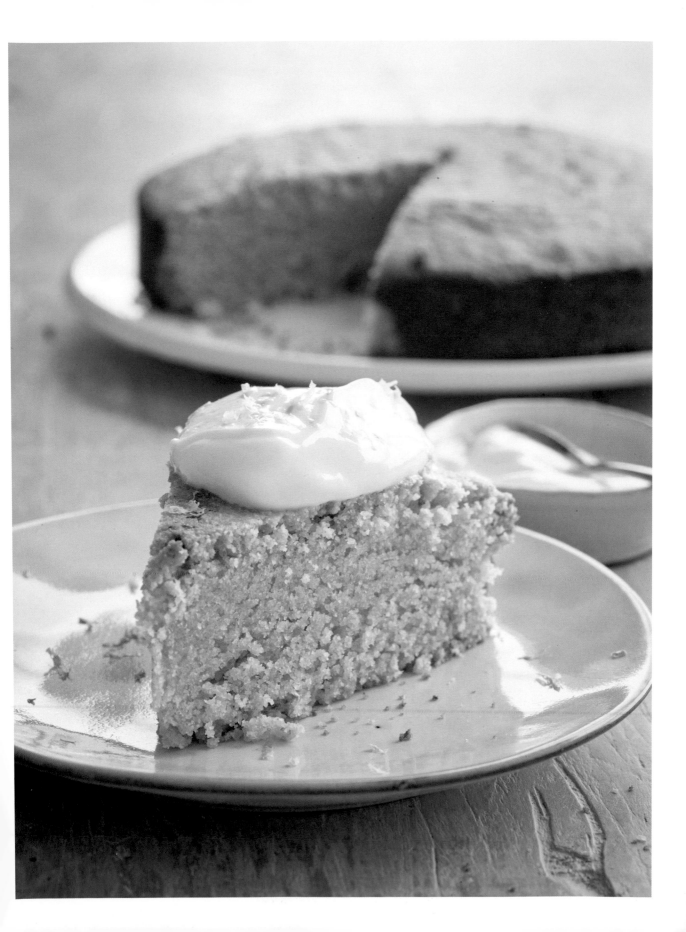

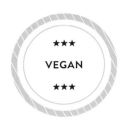

Another instant ice cream favourite. The matcha powder adds some colour and a little extra health kick, but it isn't essential so don't worry if you don't have any to hand. We love how the green of the toasted pistachios matches the creamy green of the avocado, but any nut will work well here.

Pistachio ice cream

// SERVES 2 //

40g raw unsalted pistachios
1 ripe avocado, chilled
1 small banana, peeled and frozen
2 tsp honey or maple syrup
1 tsp matcha powder (optional)
¼ tsp vanilla extract
¼ tsp lime juice
pinch sea salt flakes

1 / Toast the pistachios in a dry pan until nice and fragrant. Let cool and roughly chop.

2 / Blitz the remaining ingredients in a food processor until smooth and creamy. Fold through most of the chopped pistachios, then serve immediately with the remaining pistachios on top.

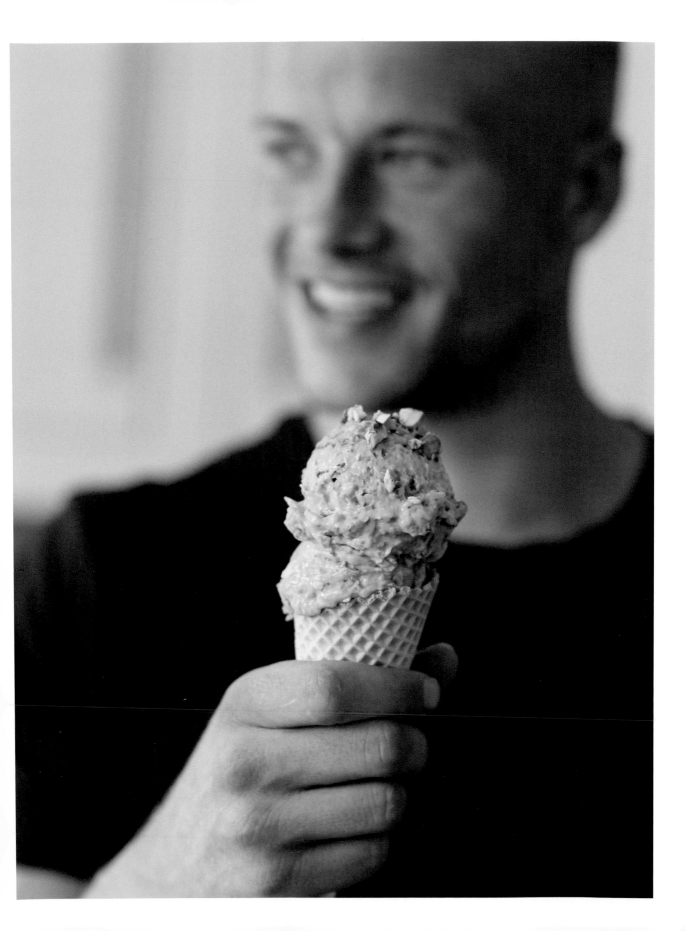

Yup, tofu in a pudding. Bear with us on this one, because it is the bomb… You're after the silken tofu here, which is often packaged in a little tetra pak and stacked down the store-cupboard aisle (as opposed to the fridge section with the firm tofu). This has the most amazing ganache texture once chilled, and we bet you no one will be able to guess what the secret ingredient is!

Chocolate orange pots

// SERVES 4 //

60g dark chocolate

½ tsp coconut oil

300g silken tofu,
   drained and excess water
   squeezed out in kitchen paper

2 tbsp maple syrup

juice and finely grated zest of
   ½ orange, plus extra shavings
   to serve

½ tsp vanilla seeds

pinch flaked sea salt

1 / Melt the chocolate and coconut oil in the microwave over medium heat for 2–3 minutes. You want the chocolate to be just melted; don't let it overcook.

2 / Put the tofu, chocolate, maple syrup, orange, vanilla and salt in the food processor and blitz until silky smooth.

3 / Pour into small glasses, jars or cups and sprinkle with the extra orange zest. Leave in the fridge to set for 2 hours.

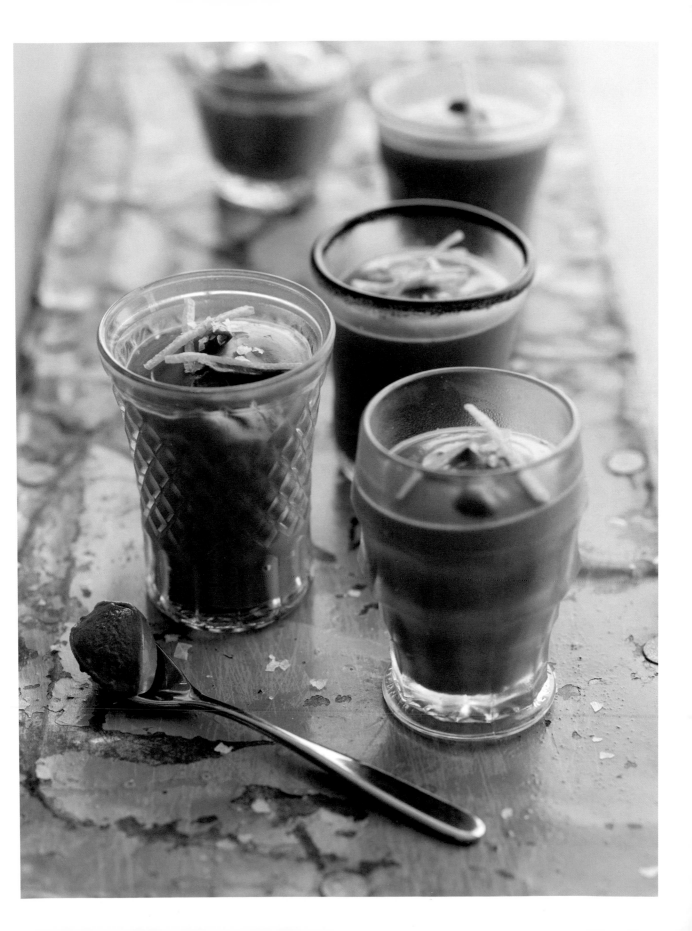

Hell yes we have a sticky toffee pudding recipe! The Pudding of all puddings, our version here is lighter and much lower in sugar than your typical stodge-fest, but no less tasty for it; just look how excited Tom is!

Sticky toffee pudding

// SERVES 6 //

150g dates
60g butter
100g coconut sugar
2 large eggs
50ml maple syrup
1 tsp bicarbonate soda
1 tsp baking powder
150g white spelt flour

SAUCE
150g dates
60g butter

1 / Preheat the oven to 180°C/Gas 4, lightly butter your baking dish.

2 / Put the dates in a bowl, cover with 150ml boiling water and leave them to soak for about 20 minutes.

3 / Put the dates and the soaking water in a food processor and blitz to a smooth purée. Transfer to a large bowl with the butter and coconut sugar and whisk together. Whisk in the eggs, one at a time, beating between each addition, followed by the maple syrup.

4 / Mix the baking powder and bicarbonate of soda with the flour in another bowl, then sift the dry ingredients into the date mixture. Using a large spoon or spatula, fold everything together until well incorporated. Pour the mixture into the prepared baking dish and bake in the oven for about 35 minutes, or until risen and a skewer inserted into the centre of the pudding comes out clean.

5 / While the sponge is cooking, make the sauce. Put the dates in a bowl and pour over 250ml boiling water. Leave to soak for about 10 minutes (you want the water to still be warm), then transfer to a food processor, add the butter and blend everything to a smooth sauce. If it's a little thick, add another splash of hot water until it is the consistency you'd like. Serve the sponge with the sauce poured over.

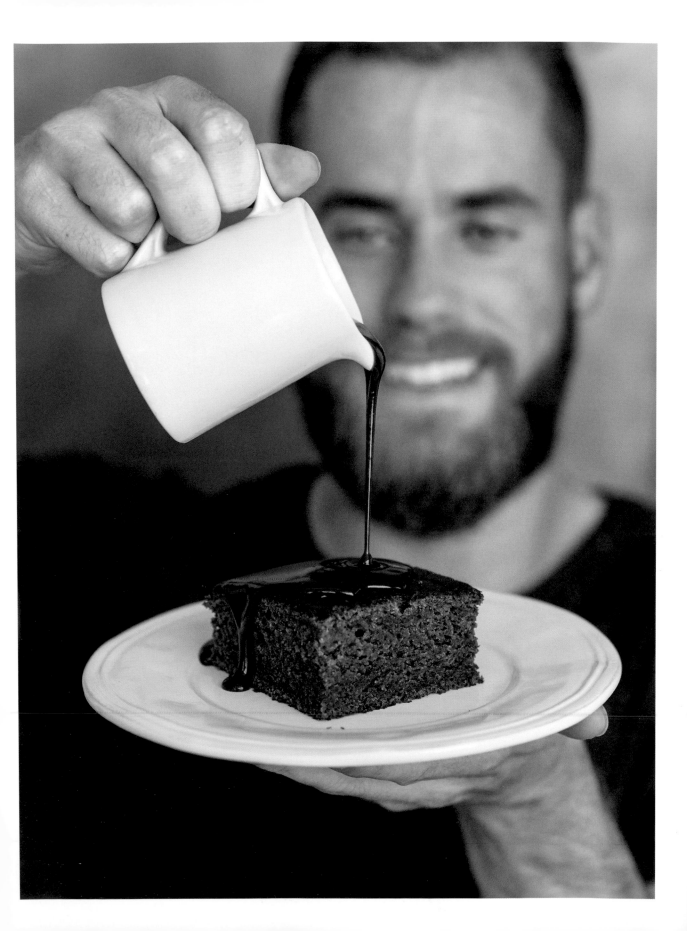

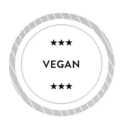

★★★
VEGAN
★★★

Another sneaky veg-cocoa combo; if you're finding the truffles a little too gooey to roll at first put the mix in the freezer for 10 minutes or so.

Avo-choc truffles

// MAKES 18–20 //

1 ripe avocado, peeled, stoned
  and roughly chopped
100g ground almonds
4½ tbsp maple syrup
50g cocoa powder, plus extra
  to roll the truffles in

1 / Put all the ingredients in a food processor and blend to form a smooth, thick paste.

2 / Sift a good layer of cocoa powder onto a plate. Scoop up small lumps of the paste and roll them between your palms to create balls. Roll the balls in the cocoa powder and store in the fridge until ready to serve.

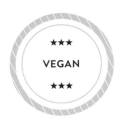

The perfect end to any roast. This version is vegan, low sugar and gluten-free depending on the oats you use; it's also warming, cinnamonny (that's a word, right?) and smells as good as it tastes. Serve with a dollop of the vanilla cream (see page 130).

Apple & blackberry crumble

// SERVES 4 //

3 apples, peeled and cut into wedges
2 tbsp runny honey
1 tsp vanilla extract
juice of 1 lemon
130g fresh or frozen blackberries

CRUMBLE TOPPING
75g coconut oil
100g oat flour
70g rolled oats
pinch sea salt
40g flaked almonds
25g ground almonds
60g brown or coconut sugar
1 tsp ground cinnamon
½ tsp mixed spice

1 / Preheat the oven to 180°C/Gas 4. Put the apples in a pan with the honey, vanilla and lemon juice. Heat over medium–low heat and cook gently for 10 minutes, until the apples are just tender. Take off the heat.

2 / Tip the apples into a baking tin and scatter with the berries.

3 / Melt the coconut oil in the microwave or in a pan. Combine with the oat flour, rolled oats, salt, flaked and ground almonds, sugar, cinnamon and mixed spice. Scatter the crumble over the top of the apples and berries.

4 / Bake in the oven for 35–45 minutes, until the juices from the fruit start to bubble up at the edges.

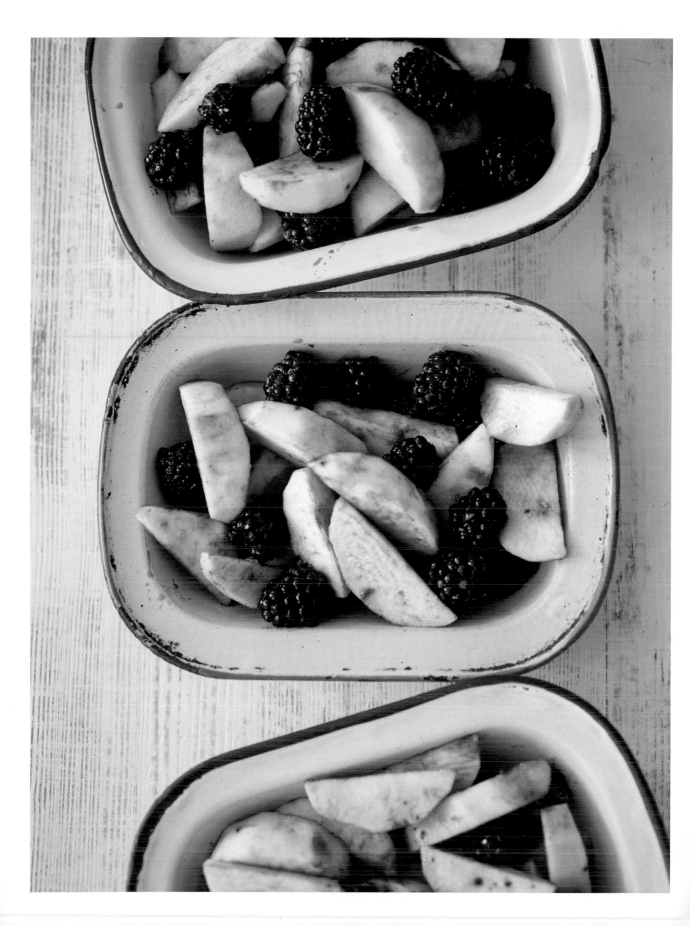

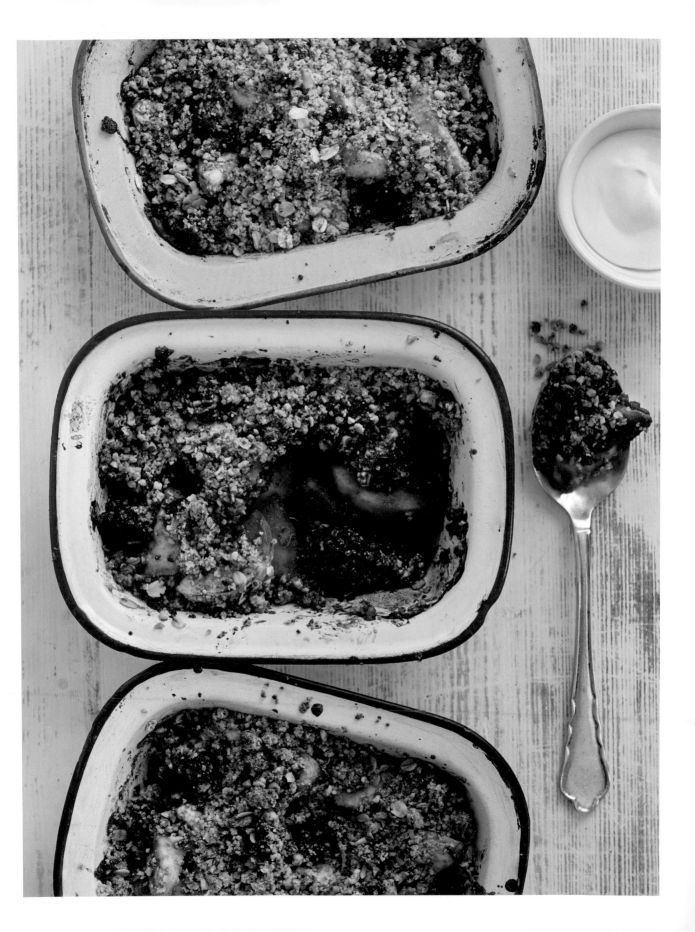

Chocolate and coconut – a match made in bounty-ful heaven. If you can't find the strong-flavoured coconut oil go with the mild stuff and simply add an extra spoonful of desiccated coconut.

Chocolate coconut cookies

||||||||||||||||||||||||||||||||||||||||||||||||||||||||||||||||||||||||||||||||||||||||

// MAKES 12 //

130g rolled oats
75g coconut oil (don't use the mild, odourless coconut oil – you want the coconut flavour in this)
1 egg
4 tbsp honey
30g cocoa powder
25g desiccated coconut
50g chocolate chips (optional)

1 / Preheat the oven to 190°C/Gas 5 and line a baking sheet with baking parchment.

2 / Put the oats in a food processor and process to grind them down to a flour. Add all the remaining ingredients, except the chocolate drops, to the food processor and blitz until well combined. Remove the blade and stir in the chocolate drops, if using.

3 / Form the dough into 12 balls by rolling portions between your palms. Place the balls on the prepared baking sheet and press down on each to form a round about 5mm thick. Bake in the oven for 15 minutes, until crisp on top but still a little gooey in the middle. Allow to cool on the baking sheet before serving.

4-ingredient heroes

The idea in this section is to take a few ingredients that you'll probably have already – butter, salt and pepper – and add just four star ingredients (hence the hero part).

This pie is a proper 'hey presto' dinner that's ready before you know it. Do use frozen veg if you have any, but beware that cutting any big florets might prove tricky!

Easy-peasy chicken pie

|||||||||||||||||||||||||||||||||||||||||||||||||||||||||||||||||||||||||||||||||||||||||||

// SERVES 4 //

800g SWEET POTATOES, peeled and cut into large chunks
40g butter
1 tbsp olive oil
6 CHICKEN THIGHS, chopped into large chunks
1 x 480g bag PREPARED VEG
jelly chicken STOCK POT
1 tbsp cornflour, dissolved in 2 tbsp water
sea salt and freshly ground black pepper

1 / Preheat the oven to 180°C/Gas 4.

2 / Boil the sweet potatoes for 12–15 minutes until tender. Tip into a colander to drain and leave for 5 minutes to steam dry. Transfer to a large mixing bowl and mash, adding the butter and a good amount of salt and pepper, then set aside.

3 / Heat the oil in a pan set over high heat and fry the chicken until browning on the outside. Meanwhile, fill a deep baking dish half full with the prepared veg. If you come across any huge florets of broccoli or cauliflower, chop those in half to speed up cooking. Tip in the browned chicken and any juices from the pan and mix together with the veg.

4 / Add the stock pot to the pan the chicken was in and top up with 450ml of boiling water. Stir over the heat until the stock cube has dissolved, then add in the cornflour and water mixture. Cook for about 5 minutes until the liquid thickens to a gravy.

5 / Pour the gravy over the chicken and veggies in the pie dish until the liquid comes to the same level as the fillings (don't add it all in if there's too much). Spoon the sweet potato mash over the top and ruffle it up a bit on the top so it's not completely smooth.

6 / Bake the pie in the oven for 40 minutes, or until the chicken and the vegetables are cooked. The sweet potato won't go brown like standard mash, but may start to blacken along the ridges where it has been ruffled up.

Full credit to Alex@thefoodgrinder for these gems. Whenever this recipe goes up on one of our accounts the response is huge; never underestimate the power of a truly fudgy brownie – particularly when you can count the ingredients on one hand.

Fudge protein brownies

||||||||||||||||||||||||||||||||||||||||||||||||||||||||||||||||||||||||||||||||||||||||||||||||

// MAKES 9 //

4 overripe BANANAS
120g crunchy PEANUT BUTTER
50g COCOA powder
30g vegan PROTEIN POWDER

1 / Preheat the oven to 180°C/Gas 4 and grease and line a 20cm square brownie tin with baking parchment.

2 / Put the bananas in a bowl and mash them to a pulp with a fork. Mix in the peanut butter, followed by the cocoa and protein powders.

3 / Spoon the batter into the prepared brownie tin, smooth level and bake for 20 minutes, until firm on top, but still fudgy and gooey in the middle. Leave to cool in the tin, then slice into 9 squares to serve.

This is such a great option for lunch or supper – quick, easy, protein-packed and delicious. Use up any leftover sweet potato wedges (see page 104), if 'leftover sweet potato wedges' isn't impossible...

Sweet potato frittata

||||||||||||||||||||||||||||||||||||||||||||||||||||||||||||||||||||||||||||||||||||||||||

// SERVES 2 //

1 tbsp olive oil
250g SWEET POTATO, peeled
  and diced into 1cm cubes
5 large EGGS
100g FETA cheese, diced into
  1cm cubes
small handful BASIL leaves,
  shredded, plus extra to serve
sea salt and freshly ground
  black pepper

1 / Preheat the grill to high.

2 / Heat the oil in a non-stick frying pan with a heatproof handle. Add the sweet potato and sauté over medium heat for 10–15 minutes until it's picked up a bit of colour on all sides and is cooked throughout. You don't have to watch this like a hawk – just remember to give it a stir every few minutes.

3 / Meanwhile, break the eggs into a mixing bowl and season with salt and pepper. Stir in the diced feta and shredded basil.

4 / Once the sweet potato is cooked, pour the egg mixture into the pan and mix around gently so that the sweet potato is spread evenly throughout. Leave the frittata to cook for about 5 minutes until the bottom is well set, then put the pan under the hot grill and cook for a further 2–3 minutes, until the top is puffing up and browned.

5 / Serve sprinkled with a little extra shredded basil.

Not just one, but *four* four-ingredient options! We do spoil you. Make these for supper and pack any leftovers up for lunch the next day.

Tart 4-ways

||||||||||||||||||||||||||||||||||||||||||||||||||||||||||||||||||||||||||

Leek, blue cheese & bacon

||||||||||||||||||||||||||||||||||||||||||||||||||||||||||||||||||||||||||

1 x 320g sheet ready rolled
  puff PASTRY
1 tbsp olive oil, plus extra
  if needed
2 small LEEKS, sliced into
  5mm thick slices
80g smoked BACON lardons
80g BLUE CHEESE, crumbled
freshly ground black pepper

1 / Preheat the oven to 200°C/Gas 6.

2 / Lay the sheet of pastry on a non-stick baking tray. On each edge of the rectangle, fold in a thin strip of pastry towards the middle, about 1cm thick, and press down gently to create a border of double-thickness pastry around the whole sheet. Prick the base in the middle several times with a fork to stop it rising up too much. Bake in the oven for 12 minutes, until beginning to turn pale golden, then remove from the oven.

3 / Meanwhile, heat the oil in a frying pan over medium heat and add the leeks and bacon. Sauté gently for about 10 minutes until the leeks are softened and just picking up some colour.

4 / Spread the cooked leeks and bacon over the pastry base, being careful not to go up onto the raised edge. Sprinkle the crumbled blue cheese over the tart and season well with pepper (you won't need salt because the bacon and cheese are both very salty). Bake for 18–20 minutes, until the pastry is cooked through and the toppings are beginning to brown.

Cream cheese, smoked salmon & spinach

||||||||||||||||||||||||||||||||||||||||||||||||||||||||||||||||||||||||

1 x 320g sheet ready-rolled
   puff PASTRY
200g baby SPINACH
150g CREAM CHEESE
100g SMOKED SALMON,
   cut into ribbons
sea salt and freshly ground
   black pepper

1 / Preheat the oven to 200°C/Gas 6.

2 / Lay the sheet of pastry on a non-stick baking tray. On each edge of the rectangle, fold in a thin strip of pastry towards the middle, about 1cm thick, and press down gently to create a border of double-thickness pastry around the whole sheet. Prick the base in the middle several times with a fork to stop it rising up too much. Bake in the oven for 12 minutes, until beginning to turn pale golden, then remove from the oven.

3 / Meanwhile, steam the spinach for 2 minutes until just wilted. Remove it from the steamer with a fork so you don't bring any water with it, lay it between several sheets of kitchen paper and gently squeeze out any excess moisture.

4 / Spread the cream cheese all over the middle of the tart, being careful not to go up onto the raised edge. Spread the cooked spinach out over that and grind over a little salt (you won't need much as the salmon will be salty) and plenty of black pepper. Sprinkle the salmon ribbons over the top of the tart. Bake for 18–20 minutes, until the pastry is cooked through and golden.

‖‖

Tomato, mozzarella & pesto

‖‖

1 x 320g sheet ready-rolled
 puff PASTRY
1 x 145g jar PESTO
2 TOMATOES (about 200g total
 weight), thinly sliced
150g MOZZARELLA cheese,
 thinly sliced
sea salt and freshly ground
 black pepper

1 / Preheat the oven to 200°C/Gas 6.

2 / Lay the sheet of pastry on a non-stick baking tray. On each edge of the rectangle, fold in a thin strip of pastry towards the middle, about 1cm thick, and press down gently to create a border of double thickness pastry around the whole sheet. Prick the base in the middle several times with a fork to stop it rising up too much. Bake in the oven for 12 minutes, until beginning to turn pale golden, then remove from the oven.

3 / Spread the pesto all over the middle of the tart, being careful not to go up onto the raised edge. Lay the tomato slices over the tart, followed by the mozzarella slices. Grind salt and pepper over the top of the tart. Bake for 18–20 minutes, until the pastry is cooked through and the cheese is beginning to brown.

Beetroot, goat's cheese & rocket

||||||||||||||||||||||||||||||||||||||||||||||||||||||||||||||||||

1 x 320g sheet ready-rolled
 puff PASTRY
150g cooked BEETROOT, grated
150g log soft GOAT'S CHEESE
25g ROCKET leaves
sea salt and freshly ground
 black pepper

1 / Preheat the oven to 200°C/Gas 6.

2 / Lay the sheet of pastry on a non-stick baking tray. On each edge of the rectangle, fold in a thin strip of pastry towards the middle, about 1cm thick, and press down gently to create a border of double-thickness pastry around the whole sheet. Prick the base in the middle several times with a fork to stop it rising up too much. Bake in the oven for 12 minutes, until beginning to turn pale golden, then remove from the oven.

3 / Meanwhile, put the grated beetroot between several sheets of kitchen paper and gently squeeze out any excess moisture. Once the pastry has come out of the oven, sprinkle the beetroot over the middle of the tart, being careful not to go up onto the raised edge. Crumble the goat's cheese all over the beetroot, season with salt and pepper, and return to the oven. Bake for 18–20 minutes, until the pastry is cooked through and the cheese is beginning to brown. Sprinkle the rocket over the tart, to serve.

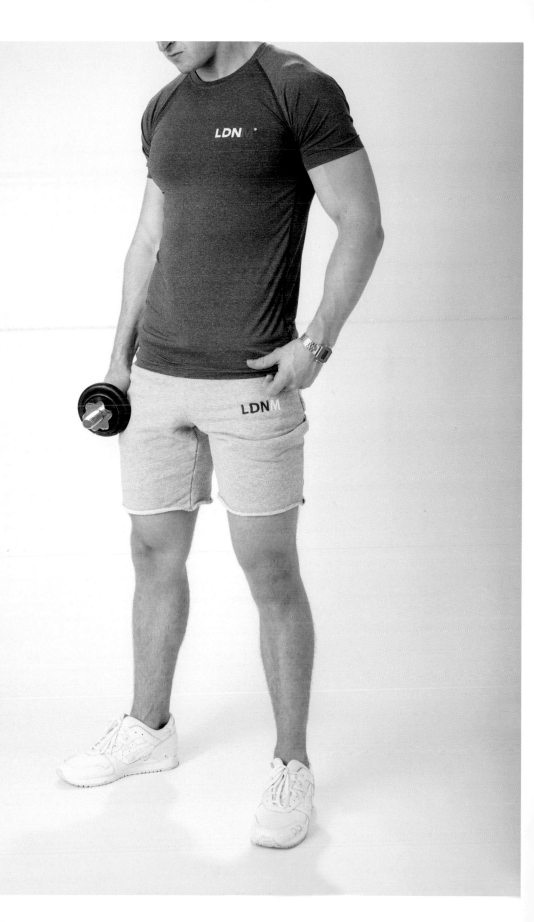

FITTER

||||||||||||||||||||||||||||||||||||||||||||||||||||||||||||||||||

If eating well is the foundation for a long-term and successful
fitness programme, then exercise provides the building blocks to
a Leaner, Fitter and Stronger you.

If you haven't exercised for a while, then the good news is that
your body craves movement and will respond very quickly to a
change in activity level. This means that, depending on how fit
you are to begin with and your body-fat percentage, you will start
seeing results fast. But just remember that you won't get super-
shredded or down to your desired weight overnight: your rate
of progress will slow down over time and might, at some point,
plateau. That's okay, in fact, that's desirable: you're more likely to
maintain your ideal physique if you get there slowly, aren't too
restrictive in your diet or too ambitious when it comes to exercise.
A diet that is too restrictive can lead to craving the 'bad' foods,
and an overambitious exercise plan can lead to burn- out, or
worse, injury.

Don't forget that maintaining your new body shape is much
easier if you make eating well and exercising well part of your
lifestyle. You're going to feel better from the inside out, move
better, and – the extra bonus that we are all aiming for – look
better too. What's not to love?

We advise a fitness programme based around two key
workouts: HIIT (high-intensity interval training) and strength
training. HIIT will improve your cardiovascular health and help
to burn fat, while strength training will improve your muscle tone
and metabolism. With a better muscle-to-fat ratio, you will burn
more calories at rest. And burning more calories at rest equals
burning more fat while at rest!

Working out from home is fine, especially as we live in
a climate that can be unpredictable, i.e., wet! But don't
underestimate the benefits of going outside and training in the
park. Even in the damp, exercising outside can lift your spirits
and bolster your mood. And then there's the competitive aspect

... continued

of training with a friend. Healthy competition is a great thing – it will spur both of you on to training better and harder, and maybe there's a cheeky pint in it for the person who's worked hardest during the week. Don't underestimate the social benefits of training at the gym. We know: the first few times that you go to the gym can be intimidating, but remember that most people are there to focus on their own work and are paying little attention to you. But working out surrounded by other people who are also working out can get you into the right mindset to train well. So whatever way you want to train – at home, the park, with a buddy or in the gym, we have the exercises for you.

MYTH BUSTING

Weights will make you bulky

Many women fear that doing weights will increase their body's bulk. In fact, weight training will not make you bulky. If your aim is to build muscle, which is a hard and lengthy process, a proper weights routine and diet will allow you to achieve this. However, incorporating weights (resistance training) into your fitness routine will not make you bulky, and is more beneficial long-term for progress and health versus cardio alone.

Weights can help benefit posture, core strength, decrease body-fat levels and increase lean muscle, strength and fitness. In older people they also help slow conditions such as weakening of the bones.

TDEE

Remember to keep an eye on your TDEE (see page 24). If you want to lose weight, make sure that you're working with a calorie deficit, but factor in your increased activity level as well. This is the same when you're working towards muscle gain. Always be aware of your increased activity levels and adjust your TDEE accordingly.

It is far better for you to opt for a calorie-controlled diet that includes the foods you enjoy – and progressive training. This means you are aware of your calorie intake while gradually increasing the intensity of your training over time.

You must do cardio every day

You do not need to do cardio every day in order to make progress. Instead, we see resistance work with supplementary cardio as the most sustainable and effective way to move towards your goals.

Performing high-intensity cardio every day will likely blunt the progress you could otherwise achieve from its inclusion in a well-structured training and nutrition routine. HIIT cardio should be used two to four times per week, depending on your ability to tolerate it.

Cardio will make you toned

The idea that cardio alone will make you toned is not entirely wrong, but spending hours tirelessly pounding away on the treadmill isn't efficient or rewarding. For fat loss, higher-intensity interval training (HIIT) and weight training is far more beneficial. And this, of course, has to be teamed with a calorie-controlled diet.

A combination of resistance training supplemented with higher and lower intensity forms of cardio is ideal to increase muscle definition. 'Toning' occurs by reducing body fat to reveal more definition of the muscle beneath the skin. This is why you can't tone a specific area like the tummy from solely completing crunches, or the back of the upper arms from only tricep kickbacks. Choosing where to lose fat from is impossible; it is only possible to reduce your total body fat level.

If you do x amount of sit ups, you will have a flat stomach – aka fat loss in a specific area through strength training

While working a specific area with resistance training may change the muscle shape, definition and size over time, it will not cause you to lose fat just from the targeted area. As previously mentioned, spot fat loss isn't possible.

If you did full-body resistance workouts and intense cardio work in combination with a calorie-controlled diet, you would have far more success in increasing overall definition than if you were to do solely donkey kickbacks, the recumbent bicycle and crunches in the pursuit of a toned bum and mid-section.

You won't get toned without supplements

Although some performance and dietary supplements are effective and useful, you can make progress towards your goals without them. While we would recommend vitamin D to most people, and additional iron supplements to women, we do not recommend any fat-burning products or thermogenic blends for one simple reason: they do not work.

Whey protein is already low-calorie and low-carbohydrate; diet whey is just an expensive gimmick. Raspberry ketones, fat burners, skinny or detox teas, carb blockers and basically any product pushed by someone off 'Desperate for Fame Island' is, in our view, a complete and utter waste of money.

" Be stronger than your excuses "

High-Intensity Interval Training (HIIT)

||||||||||||||||||||||||||||||||||||||||||||||||||||

High-intensity interval training, or HIIT, is the best way to get your heart rate up and burn more fat less amount of time. The idea is simple: short bursts of activity, giving it 100 per cent, alternated with slightly longer rest periods. HIIT is so effective because you are doing a lot of hard work in a very short period of time. This burns a lot of calories and because you are working in an anaerobic state (without enough oxygen), it builds up an oxygen deficit. This oxygen deficit causes your cells to adapt, increasing your fitness and also burning calories for up to 48 hours afterwards.

It's an incredibly efficient way of exercising and its effects are long-lasting – after a session of HIIT, your body will burn more calories for up to 48 hours. Moderate cardio isn't anywhere near as efficient, takes more time to do and doesn't burn as much fat.

5 BENEFITS OF HIIT

- It's a great workout in only a short time, and you only need to do it 2–4 times per week: perfect to fit in around your busy lifestyle
- Ideal for losing fat and maintaining muscle mass
- Excellent for your cardiovascular health
- Boosts endurance
- Always challenging – HIIT never gets easier, you just get better and can push yourself harder

HOW OFTEN?

HIIT is, as its name states, high-intensity. If you do too many HIIT sessions a week, you run a real risk of overtraining. Overtraining can increase the risk of injury and burnout. We recommend doing HIIT two to four times a week, depending on your tolerance for it.

" If it doesn't challenge you... it doesn't change you "

HIIT WORKOUTS

|||||||||||||||||||||||||||||

HIIT WORKOUT 1
STATIC BIKE PYRAMID
start and finish with a
3-minute low-resistence
warm up/down.

The red blocks represent your
exertion period, the blue are
your rests.

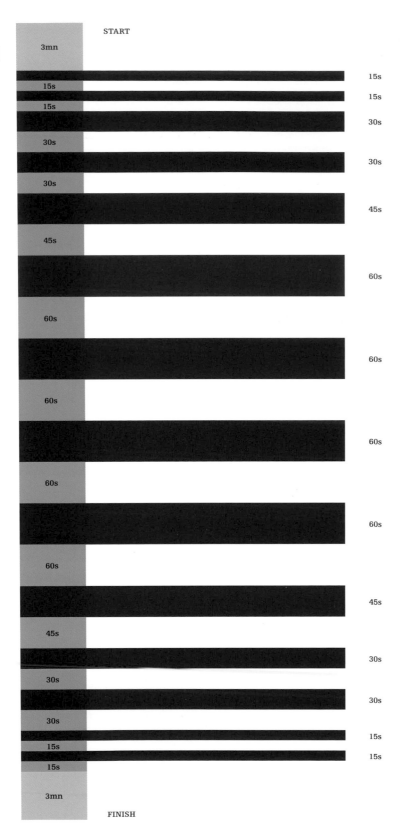

HIIT WORKOUT 2
CROSS-TRAINER

Start and finish with a
3-minute low resistance
warm up/down.

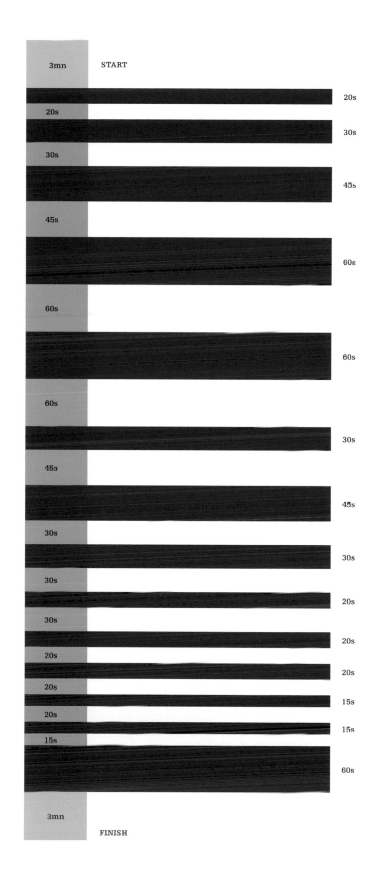

HIIT WORKOUT 3
TREADMILL

Start and finish with
a 3-minute low-speed
warm up/down.

*Note that between each set, you should
hold both handles and place one leg on
each side of the treadmill, allowing the
belt to continue to rotate. Ensure you use
the safety clip and match your leg speed
to the treadmill before getting back on.*

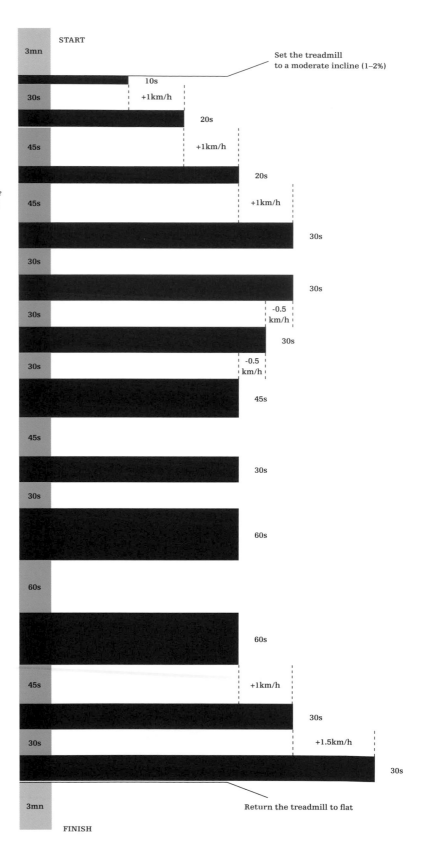

Set the treadmill
to a moderate incline (1–2%)

START

3mn

10s
30s   +1km/h

20s
45s   +1km/h

20s
45s   +1km/h

30s
30s

30s
30s

-0.5
km/h
30s   30s

-0.5
km/h
30s   45s

45s   30s

30s   60s

60s   60s

45s   +1km/h

30s
30s   +1.5km/h

30s

3mn   Return the treadmill to flat

FINISH

HIIT WORKOUT 4
ROWING

Start and finish with
a 3-minute low-resistance
warm up/down.

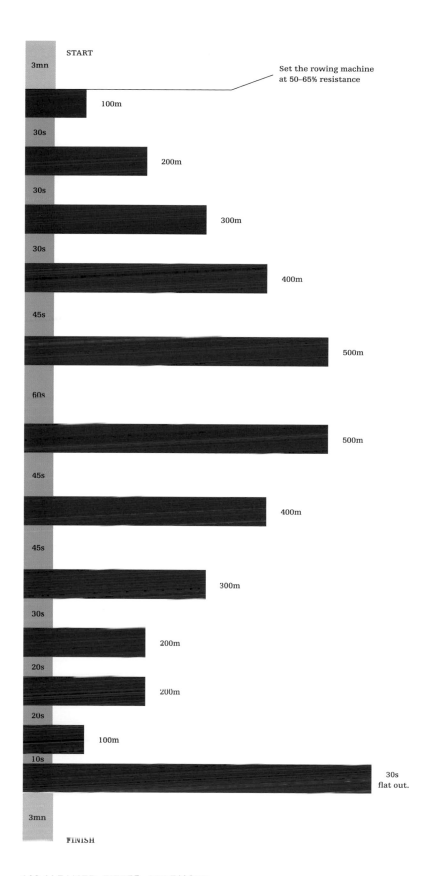

START

Set the rowing machine
at 50–65% resistance

3mn

100m

30s

200m

30s

300m

30s

400m

45s

500m

60s

500m

45s

400m

45s

300m

30s

200m

20s

200m

20s

100m

10s

30s
flat out.

3mn

FINISH

HIIT WORKOUT 5
SWIMMING

Start and finish with 2 easy lengths of any stroke of choice.

We recommend doing the sprints front crawl. But please use the stroke you feel most comfortable doing.

WATER SPRINTS

Head to the deep end. Mimic sprinting in the water, either static or moving forwards.

FINISHERS

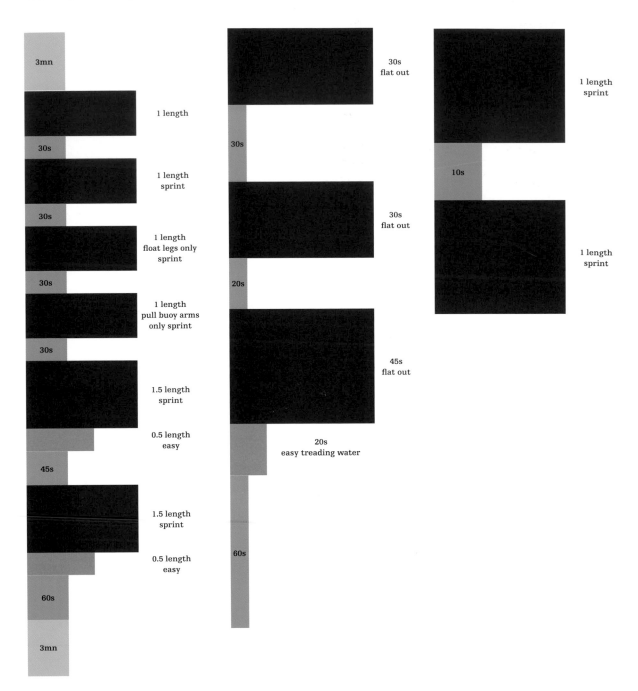

3mn	
	1 length
30s	
	1 length sprint
30s	
	1 length float legs only sprint
30s	
	1 length pull buoy arms only sprint
30s	
	1.5 length sprint
	0.5 length easy
45s	
	1.5 length sprint
	0.5 length easy
60s	
3mn	

WATER SPRINTS

	30s flat out
30s	
	30s flat out
20s	
	45s flat out
	20s easy treading water
60s	

FINISHERS

	1 length sprint
10s	
	1 length sprint

Tabata circuits

||||||||||||||||||||||||||||||||||||||||||||||||||

Tabata comprises 8 x 20-second intervals
followed by a 10-second rest. Here are five
Tabata-style circuits using four different
exercises. You simply perform the four exercises
consecutively for two rounds, to complete the
intervals. We find this way increases variety and
prevents the workout from becoming boring.

" The only
workout
you regret
is the one
you didn't do... "

Circuit 1

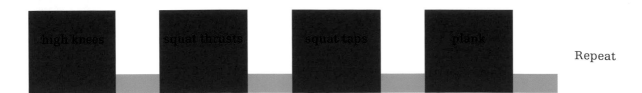

high knees squat thrusts squat taps plank

Repeat

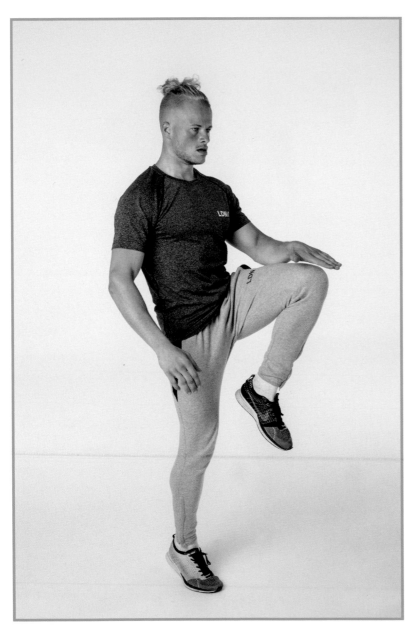

HIGH KNEES

With you elbows by your side, hold your hands out directly in front of you.

Begin running on the spot, keeping your arms and hands in place.

While running, aim to touch your knees to the palms of your hands by lifting your legs high with each stride.

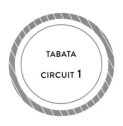

SQUAT THRUSTS

Assume a press-up position, hands shoulder width apart.

Simultaneously jump your feet towards your hands – tucking the knees under the torso – before jumping back to the start.

Repeat at a fast pace.

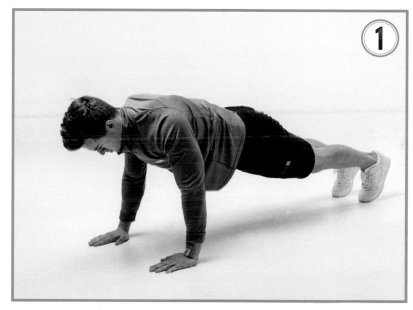

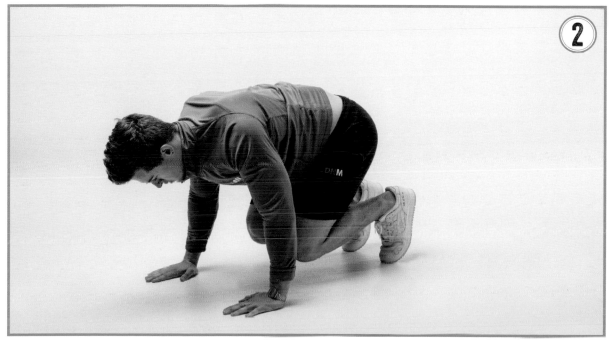

SQUAT TAPS

Start in a regular squat position.

Explosively jump upwards, move your feet to the middle of your body, landing on the balls of your feet with soft knees.

Without allowing your heels to touch the floor, jump your feet outwards to the starting position, lowering to the base of the squat and repeating.

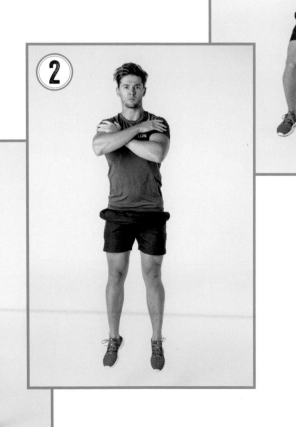

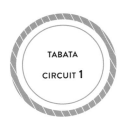
PLANK

Place your forearms flat on the floor with your elbows just within, and directly below, your shoulders.

Your body should be in a straight line from head to toe, with your neck neutral.

Keep your core tight throughout and your breathing regular.

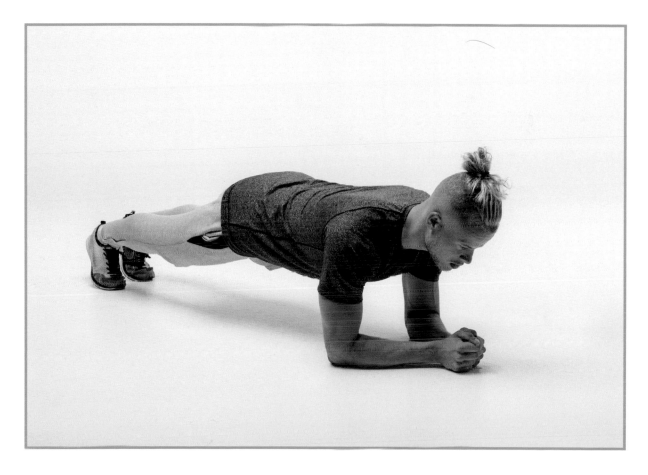

Circuit 2

||||||||||||||||||||||||||||||||||||||||||||

squat jumps · mountain climbers · commandos · lying leg raises · Repeat

SQUAT JUMPS

Stand with your feet shoulder width apart. Your body position and movement should be the same as if you were performing a regular squat, however on the upward phase, jump explosively upwards as high as you can.

Land with soft knees and repeat.

Keep your head looking forwards throughout.

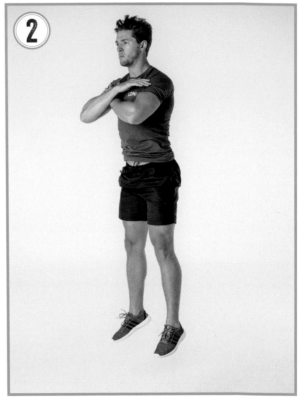

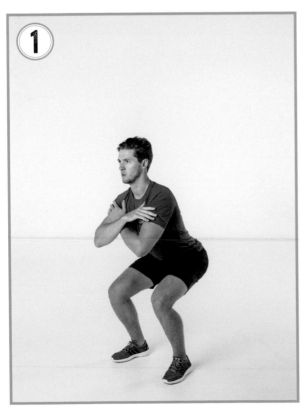

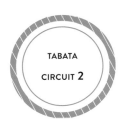
MOUNTAIN CLIMBER

Assume a press-up position
and draw one knee under your
body (directly forwards) as far
as comfortably possible.

Return to the starting position
and repeat with the opposite
leg.

Draw you knee towards the
opposite elbow to increase the
difficulty.

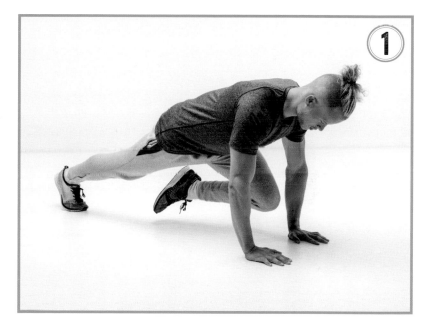

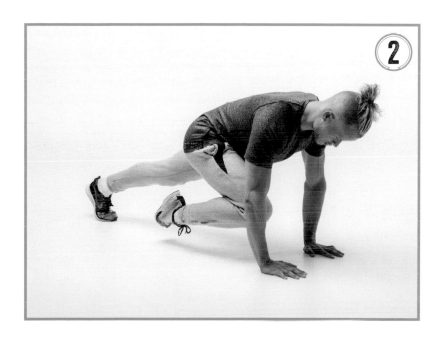

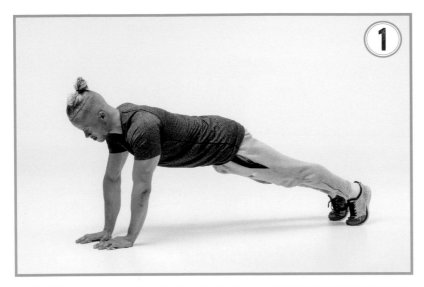

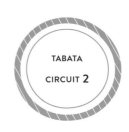

COMMANDO

Start in a regular plank position, and move to the peak of a press-up position, one arm at a time.

Lower into a plank position one arm at a time.

Keep the core tight throughout; to prevent lateral and vertical movement.

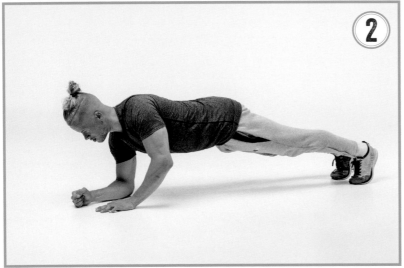

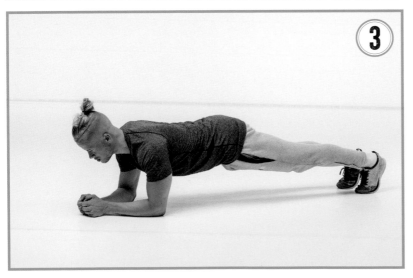

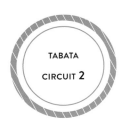

LYING LEG RAISES

Lie flat on a mat with your arms by your side, or beneath the bum if this is more comfortable.

Lift your feet upwards until the feet are directly above the hips, keeping the legs straight.

In a controlled manner return to the starting position, but do not allow your feet to touch the mat.

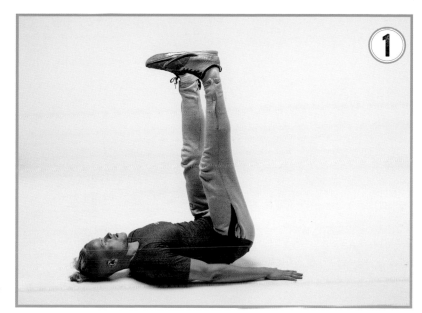

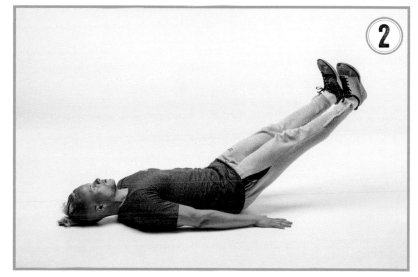

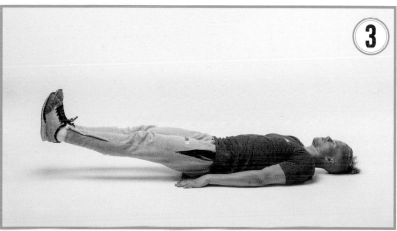

Circuit 3

Repeat

STEP UPS

Take a bench and place your leading foot on it, torso leant forwards and then drive through your front leg. Bring yourself up to a standing position on the bench.

Lower yourself in a controlled manner and land softly.

Reset and repeat the movement.

RUSSIAN TWISTS

Lie down on the floor and raise your back and legs to form a v-shape, keeping your back straight, your knees bent and your feet on the floor.

Pick up your weight and lower it to each side, left and right, turning with your weight as you go and looking in the direction of the turn.

To challenge yourself, raise your feet off the ground, keeping the v-shape.

STAR JUMPS

Stand tall with your hands by your side, before jumping both feet outwards and simultaneously moving the hands away from the body to head height.

Land softly, before jumping back to the start position.

Repeat at a fast pace.

BENT OVER ROW

With soft knees and your torso leant forwards, keep the back flat throughout.

Take a shoulder width overhand grip and draw the bar into your belly button, keeping the elbows close past the sides.

Slowly lower to the base of the rep, feeling a stretch through the back before repeating.

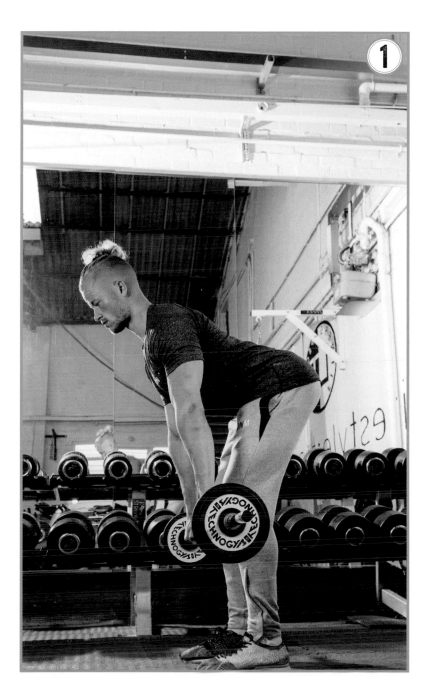

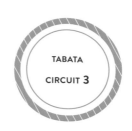

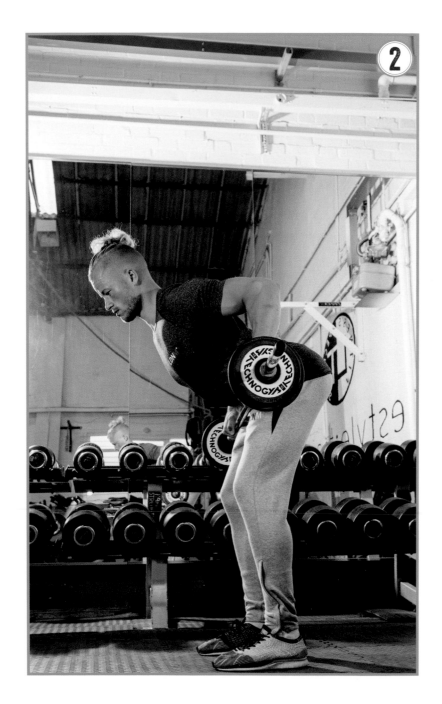

Circuit 4

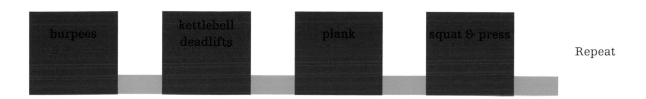

| burpees | kettlebell deadlifts | plank | squat & press | Repeat |

BURPEES

Assume a press-up position and jump both feet in, tucking the knees under the torso, before jumping vertically and extending the body.

Land softly and place the hands in the same position, before jumping the feet back out to a start position.

Repeat at a fast pace.

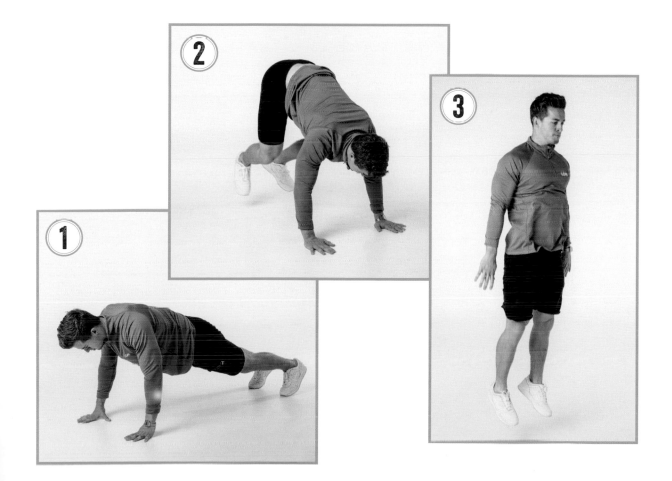

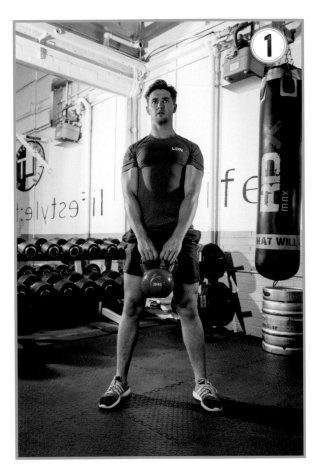

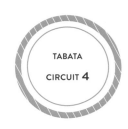
KETTLEBELL DEADLIFT

Set your feet shoulder width apart, toes angled forward or slightly outwards.

Assume the base of a deadlift position with the kettlebell directly between the mid-foot touching the floor.

Bend at your knees and hips, and keep your back straight. Grasp the handle. Drive upwards, extending your body and pulling your shoulders back at the top of the rep.

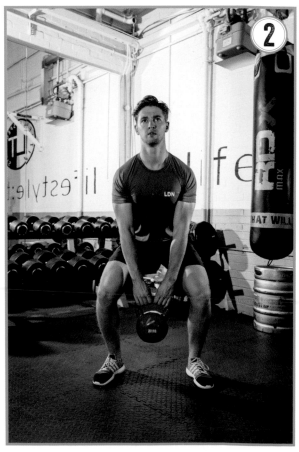

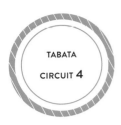
PLANK

Place your forearms flat on the floor with your elbows just within and directly below your shoulders.

Your body should be in a straight line from head to toe with your neck neutral.

Keep your core tight throughout and your breathing regular.

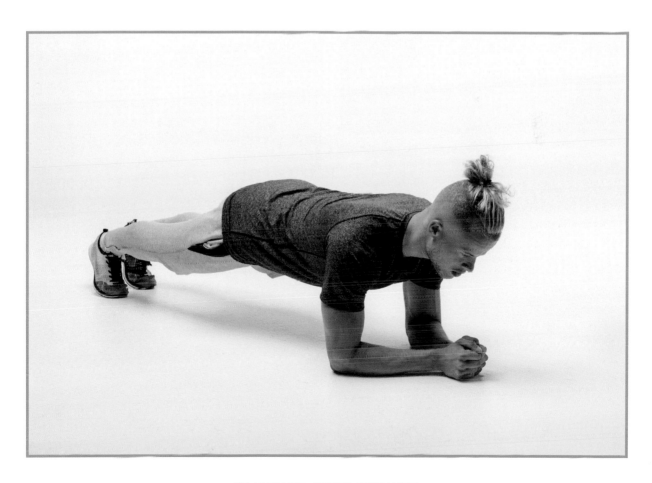

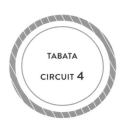
SQUAT AND PRESS

Place your feet shoulder width apart, with your back straight and your head neutral/looking forwards throughout.

Grip the dumbbells at shoulder height and squat as low as comfortable, before standing tall and pressing the dumbbells overhead.

Lower them to the shoulders and repeat.

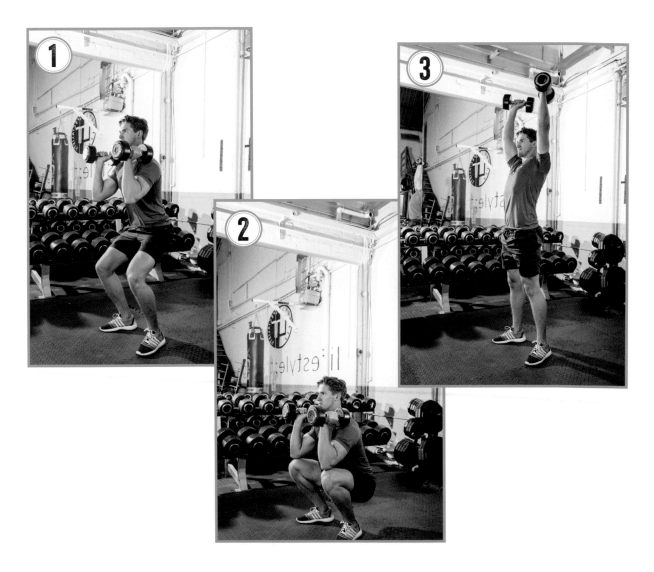

Circuit 5

||||||||||||||||||||||||||||||||||||||||||||

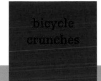 squat taps

bicycle crunches

military press

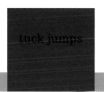 tuck jumps

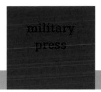

Repeat

SQUAT TAPS

Start in a regular squat position.

Explosively jump upwards, move your feet to the middle of your body and land on the balls of your feet with soft knees.

Without allowing your heels to touch the floor, jump your feet outwards to the starting position. Lower to the base of the squat and repeat.

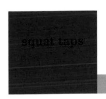

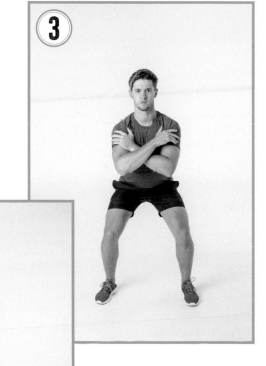

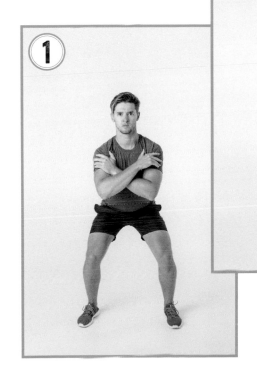

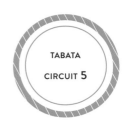

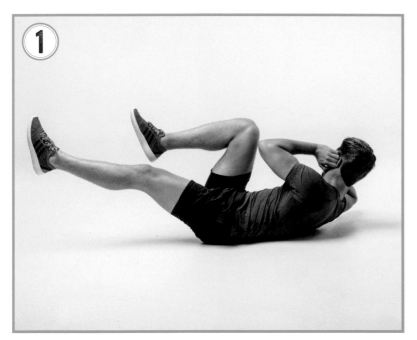

BICYCLE CRUNCHES

Lie flat on a mat, hands touching your head and knees bent so that your lower legs are parallel to the floor.

Crunch one shoulder towards the opposite knee, extending the other leg away from you.

Return to the starting position and repeat for the opposite side.

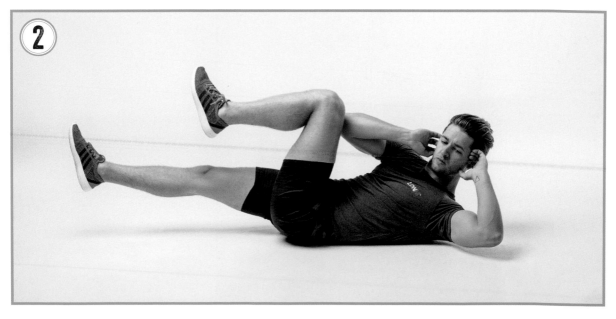

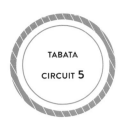

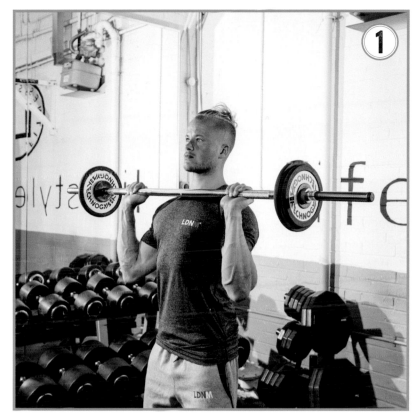

MILITARY PRESS

Place your feet slightly wider than shoulder width apart (staggered if preferred).

Grip the bar, hands shoulder width apart, or slightly wider; start with it touching your chest just below your collarbone.

Press upwards, stopping just before full extension of your elbows. Control the return phase.

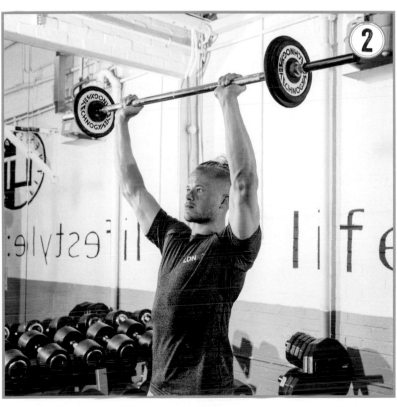

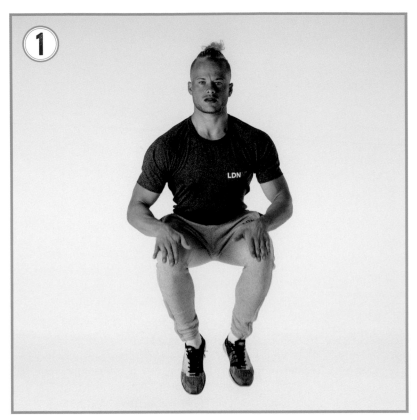

TUCK JUMPS

Assume the top of a squat position, before sinking slightly and jumping powerfully upwards.

Tuck the knees up and into the chest in flight, before landing with soft knees in the start position.

Repeat at a comfortable pace.

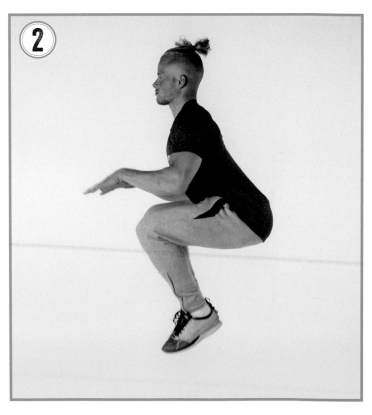

Gym-free workouts

||||||||||||||||||||||||||||||||||||||||||||||||||||||||

Free, convenient – sometimes there's no beating
the great outdoors (and indoors for that matter!).

In the next few sections we'll introduce you to some new terms;
they may already be familiar, or completely alien - either way they
will definitely take your workout to the next level.

DROP SET

A drop set is where you perform the exercise
with a heavy weight for X number of reps, then
reduce the weight by around 30–40% before
completing Y more reps with no rest between
the heavy and light sets. This method of training
will cause a burning feeling in your muscles but
ensures you use more of the target muscle fibres,
which equals more calories burnt!

SUPERSET

A superset is two different exercises performed
back to back, with no rest between the two –
completing the assigned number of reps on the
first exercise before immediately moving on to
the second exercise. A superset can be performed
on the same body part, or on two differing body
parts. This type of training can be used to save
time, recruit more muscle fibres and simply to
add variation.

6–12–25

This is a great way to work varying rep ranges
and perform a lot of work quickly and brutally!
It can be used on one muscle group or in pairs
with a main and secondary muscle group.

You should start with a big compound
exercise, performing 6 reps with a 4-second
eccentric (downwards) movement. Immediately
move on to another big, but less taxing, exercise,
performing 12 reps with 3-second eccentric
phases. Lastly you finish with 25 reps on an
isolation exercise, with 1–2 second eccentric
phases for a killer burn. Make sure you don't
rest between the exercises!

Workout 1 Park Bench

||||||||||||||||||||||||||||||||||||||||||||||||||||||||||||||||||||||||||||||||||

You will need a sturdy park bench (make sure it's not a memorial one!).

EXERCISE 1:
SINGLE-LEG STEP UP

Take a bench and place your leading foot on it, torso leant forwards and then drive through your front leg. Bring yourself up to a standing position on the bench.

Lower yourself in a controlled manner and land softly.

Reset and repeat the movement.

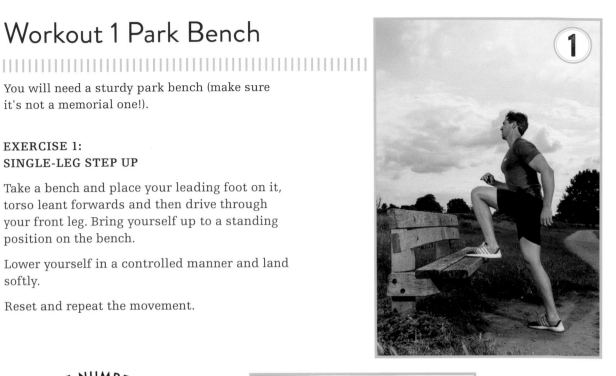

THE NUMBERS

10	**30** s	3
REPEATS	**REST**	**SETS**
switch legs		

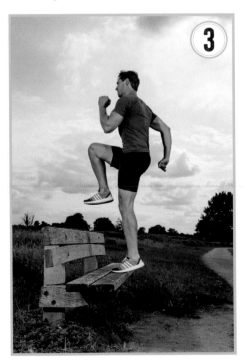

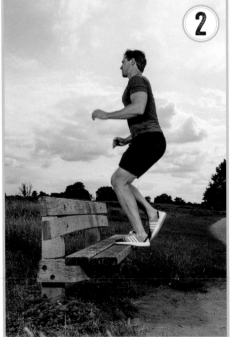

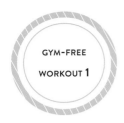

THE NUMBERS

10	30 s	3
REPEATS	REST	SETS

EXERCISE 2:
BENCH DIPS

With your body in front of a bench, take a narrow grip behind you.

Keep your elbows tucked in throughout and your body upright. Lower yourself down until your elbows hit 90 degrees, then push upwards, stopping just prior to locking out your elbows.

Prevent the elbows flaring outwards.

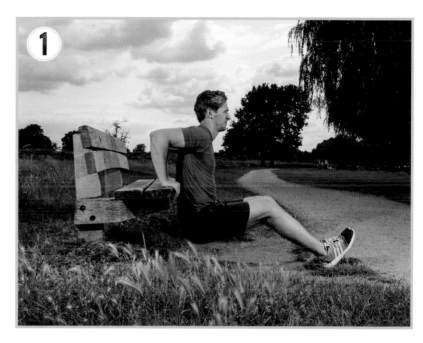

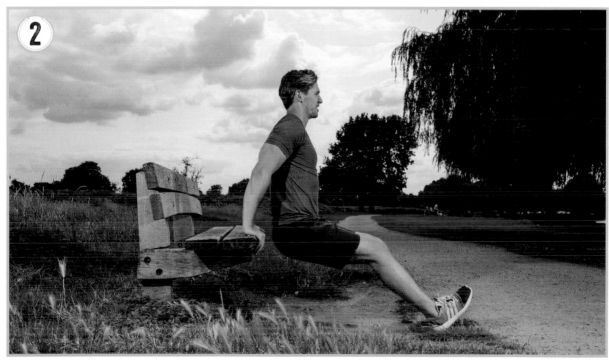

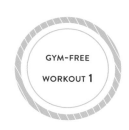
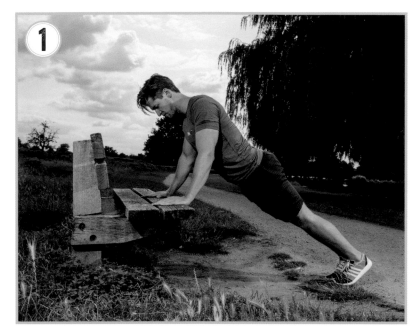

EXERCISE 3:
BENCH PRESS UPS

Assume a normal press-up position (see page 212), with the hands raised on a bench.

Lower the chest to touch the bench, before driving the body away and keeping the core tight.

Control the movement and repeat.

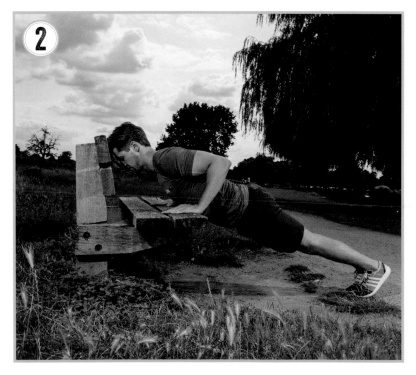

THE NUMBERS

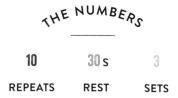

10	**30** s	3
REPEATS	REST	SETS

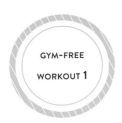

THE NUMBERS

30	**30**s	**3**
INTERVALS	REST	SETS

EXERCISE 4:
MOUNTAIN CLIMBERS (HANDS RAISED)

Assume a press-up position (with the hands raised on the bench) and draw one knee under your body (directly forwards) as far as comfortably possible.

Return to the starting position and repeat with the opposite leg.

Draw you knee towards the opposite elbow to increase the difficulty.

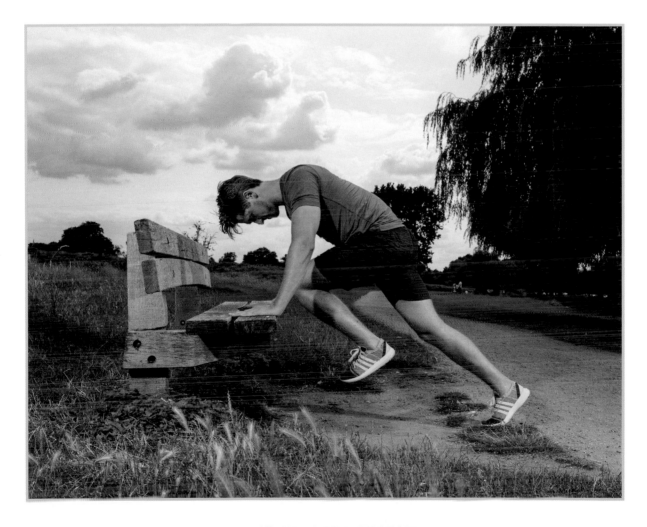

Workout 2 Outdoors

|||||||||||||||||||||||||||||||||||||||||||||||||||||||||||||||||

Find a relatively large space with no obstacles. Mark your start point with a leaf, stone, piece of clothing or other visible marker. Walk 100 strides and mark this point too. Return to your start point.

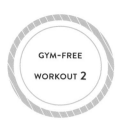

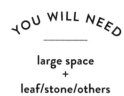

YOU WILL NEED

large space
+
leaf/stone/others

EXERCISE 1:
SQUAT JUMPS SUPERSET TO PRESS UPS

Stand with your feet shoulder width apart. Your body position and movement should be same as if you were performing a regular squat, however on the upward phase, jump explosively upwards as high as you can.

Land with soft knees and repeat.

Keep your head looking forwards throughout.

//

Start with your hands slightly wider than your shoulders, arms fully extended.

Focus on keeping your body flat throughout the rep. Your elbows should stay close to your body, your chin almost touching the ground at the bottom of each rep. Push your body upwards.

Avoid locking out your elbows at the peak of the rep.

THE NUMBERS

15/15	45 s	4
REPEAT/S	REST	ROUNDS

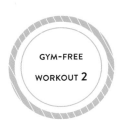

EXERCISE 2:
COMMANDOS SUPERSET TO ALTERNATING LUNGES

Start in a regular plank position and move to the peak of a press-up position one arm at a time.

Lower into a plank position one arm at a time.

Keep the core tight throughout, preventing lateral and vertical movement.

//

Stand upright with your arms by your sides.

Step forwards, landing with a slight bend at your knee. Control the eccentric phase until your front knee is at a right angle (knee directly above ankle).

From here drive up and step back through your front leg to a standing position and repeat for the other leg.

THE NUMBERS

20/30	45 s	4
REPEAT/S	REST	ROUNDS

EXERCISE 3:
STEP UPS SUPERSET TO BICYCLE CRUNCHES

Take a bench and place your leading foot on it, torso leant forwards and then drive through your front leg. Bring yourself up to a standing position on the bench.

Lower yourself in a controlled manner and land softly.

Reset and repeat the movement.

//

Lie flat on a mat, hands touching your head and feet raised from the floor and a 90-degree angle at your knees/hips.

Crunch one shoulder towards the opposite knee, extending the other leg away from you.

Return to the starting position and repeat for the opposite side.

THE NUMBERS

20/30	30 s	5
REPEAT/S	REST	ROUNDS

EXERCISE 4: STATIC LUNGES / SQUATS / GLUTE BRIDGES

Static lunge

Stand with one foot forward and the other back, making a triangle with your legs. Without moving your feet, lower your rear leg until your knee almost touches the floor while bending your front leg, then repeat with your other side.

Squats

Stand tall with the feet outside shoulder width.

With your weight through the heels, sink down until your thighs are parallel with the ground.

Press evenly through the feet; driving up to standing whilst keeping the back straight and knees from caving inward.

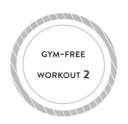

GYM-FREE

WORKOUT 2

THE NUMBERS

20s	10s	3
INTERVALS	REST	SETS

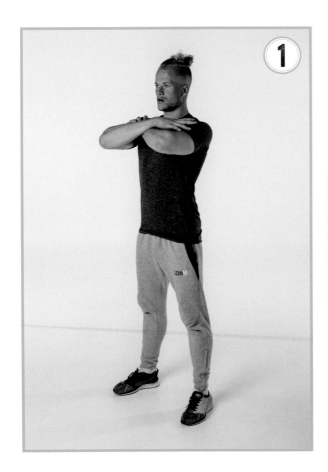

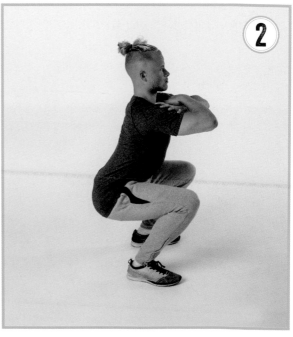

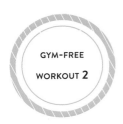

Glute bridges

Lie on your back with the feet drawn towards the glutes, just outside shoulder width.

Extend the hips to form a straight line between your knees and shoulders by driving the bum upwards.

Lower slowly, touch the floor and repeat.

" Focus on yourself, not others "

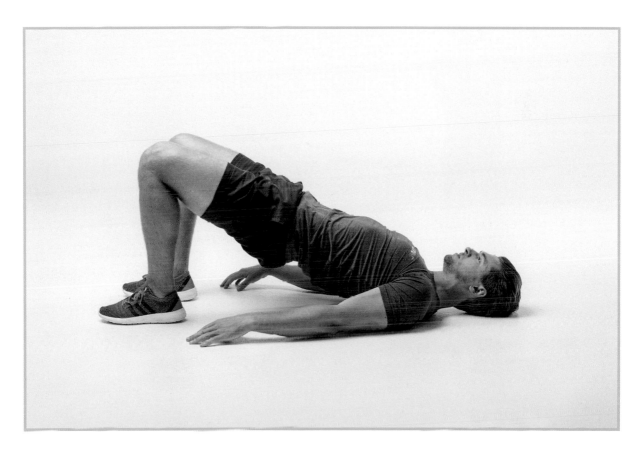

Workout 3 Sofa workout

||||||||||||||||||||||||||||||||||||||||||||||||||||||||||||||||||||||||||||||

Sofas are good for many things – watching Netflix on, napping on, eating noodles on – but contrary to their sit-soft reputation, they also make an excellent workout tool.

THE NUMBERS

12-15	30 s	4
REPEAT	REST	SETS

EXERCISE 1: FEET RAISED CRUNCHES

Lie on a mat with your legs at a 90-degree angle to your body, feet placed on top of a sofa.

Shuffle your body so that your bum is close to the sofa and there is a 90-degree angle at your knees.

Keep your neck neutral and crunch directly up, pause for a second before slowly returning to the start.

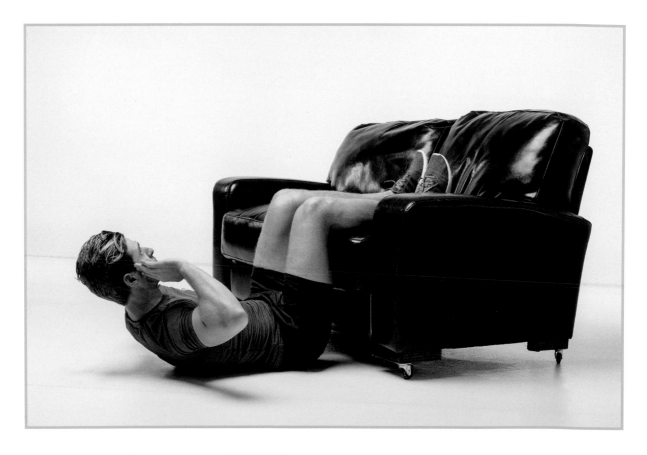

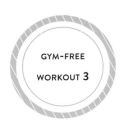

EXERCISE 2: SOFA DIPS

With your body in front of a sofa, take a narrow grip, behind you.

Keep your elbows tucked in throughout and your body upright, lower yourself down until your elbows hit 90 degrees, then push upwards, stopping just prior to locking out your elbows.

Prevent the elbows flaring outwards.

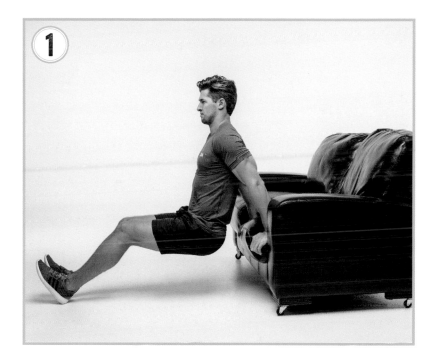

THE NUMBERS

10-12	30s	3
REPEATS	REST	SETS

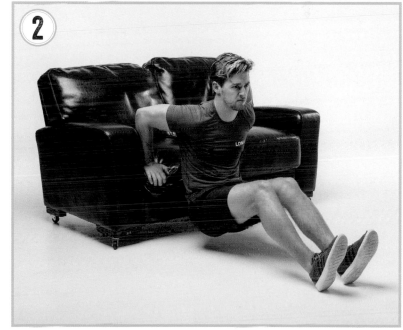

EXERCISE 3:
MOUNTAIN CLIMBERS (HANDS RAISED)

Assume a press-up position with the hands raised and draw one knee under your body (directly forwards) as far as comfortably possible.

Return to the starting position and repeat with the opposite leg.

Draw your knee towards the opposite elbow to increase the difficulty.

THE NUMBERS

30s	**20**s	4
INTERVALS	REST	SETS

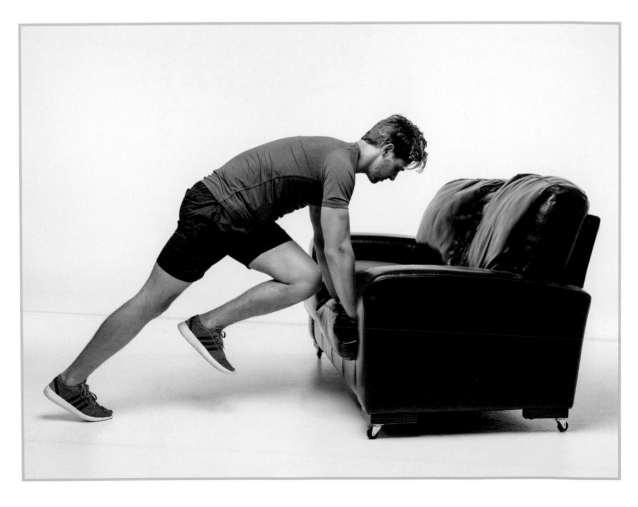

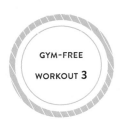
EXERCISE 4:
SOFA CRUNCHES

Perch yourself on the edge of the sofa and lift your feet off the floor.

Keeping your core strong, crunch your body and knees together while maintaining balance on the edge of the sofa.

Hold this for a second before extending your body and legs back to the starting position and repeat without allowing your feet to touch the floor.

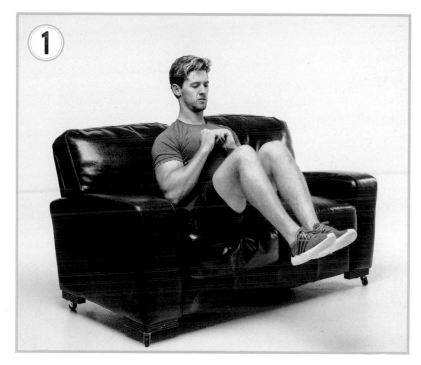

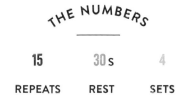

THE NUMBERS

15	**30** s	**4**
REPEATS	REST	SETS

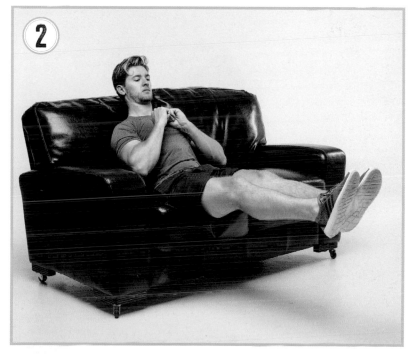

Buddy training

||||||||||||||||||||||||||||||||||||||||||||||||||

A bit of a competitive spirit can go a long way! Find a buddy on the same level as you and egg each other on to improve your fitness levels. Another advantage of training with a buddy is that they can chivvy you up on days when you're not feeling like working out – and you can do the same for them, of course!

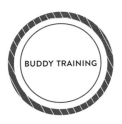

BUDDY TRAINING

PRESS-UP CHALLENGE

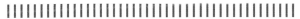

Keep the same technique as explained on page 212.

Perform alternate press ups with your partner until one of you can perform no more.

When one of you fails, rest for 45 seconds before repeating – winner is the best of 3!

THE NUMBERS

3	45 s	3
BEST OF	REST	SETS

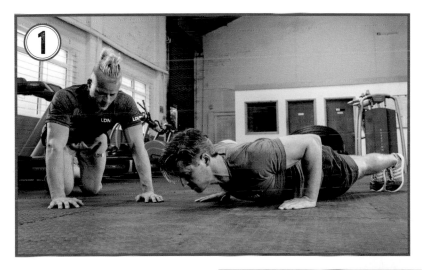

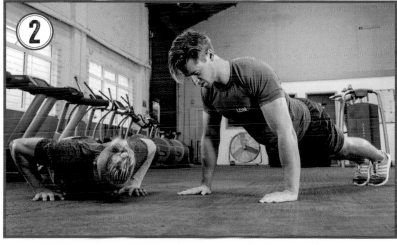

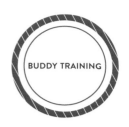

THE NUMBERS

3   **45**s   3

BEST OF   REST   SETS

PLANK CHALLENGE

||||||||||||||||||||||||||||||||||||||||||

Perform a plank with the same technique as previously explained.

Both of you should hold the plank for as long as possible until one of you has to stop.

When one of you fails, rest for 45 seconds before repeating – winner is the best of 3!

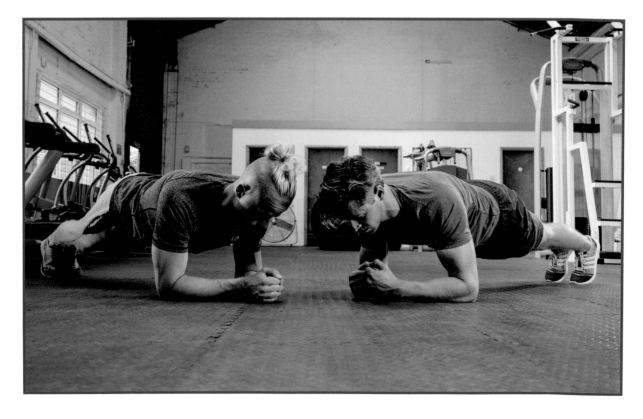

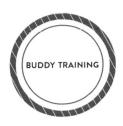

SIT UPS PASSING MEDICINE BALL

||||||||||||||||||||||||||||||

With a partner link your feet at the ankles and assume a sit up position.

With one person holding the ball to their chest, simultaneously sit up together and pass the ball, before returning to the base of the rep.

Aim to stay in time and keep passing the ball. When one of you fails, rest for 45 seconds before repeating – winner is the best of 3!

THE NUMBERS

3	45 s	3
BEST OF	REST	SETS

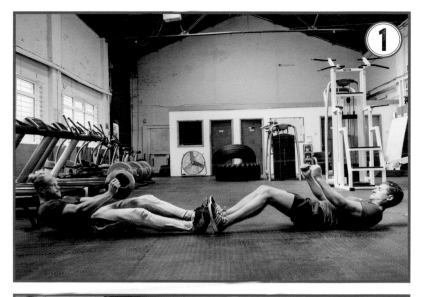

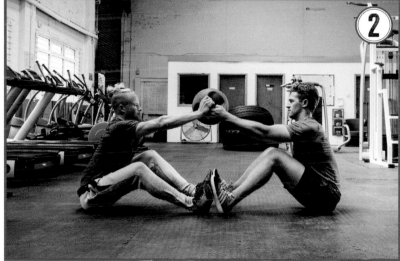

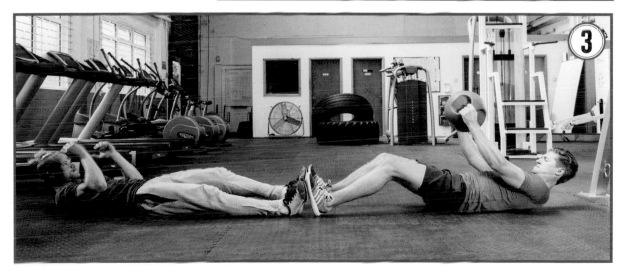

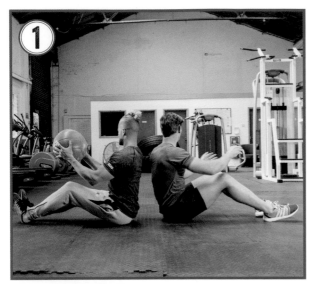

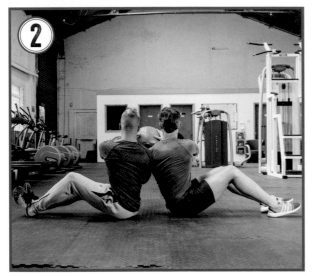

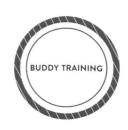

RUSSIAN TWIST AND PASS

||||||||||||||||||||||||||||||||||||||||||||||

Sit back to back with your partner. One of you hold the medicine ball and twist to your right.

The other partner should twist to the left to meet the pass of the medicine ball, then twist to the other side, where the original partner takes back the ball.

Aim to stay in time and keep passing the medicine ball around you. When one of you fails, rest for 45 seconds before repeating. Make sure to switch directions between sets. Winner is the best of 3!

THE NUMBERS

3	45s	3
BEST OF	REST	SETS

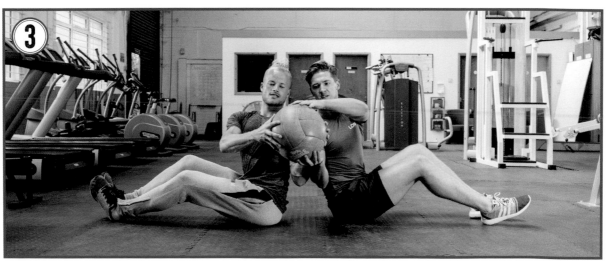

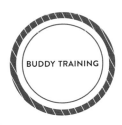
MEDICINE BALL SLAM PASSES

||||||||||||||||||||||||||||||||

One partner throws the medicine ball down and at an angle; the other partner catches and returns the slam so their partner can catch.

Repeat.

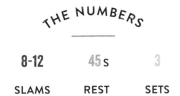

THE NUMBERS

8-12	45 s	3
SLAMS	REST	SETS

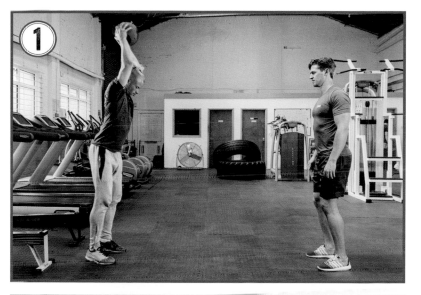

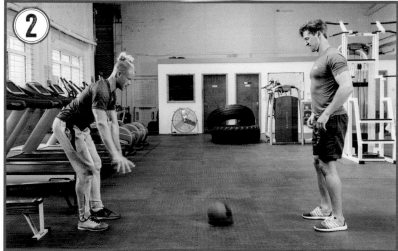

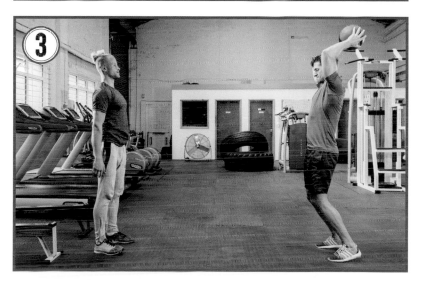

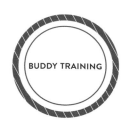

SHUTTLE RUNS, TAG & GO

||||||||||||||||||||||||||||||||||||||||||||

Stand about 25 meters away from each other and use a water bottle to mark your starting positions.

Sprint to your buddy and back to your starting position; your partner sprints when you're back at your starting position.

Your rest is your partner's sprint period.

THE NUMBERS

6-10	30 s	3
50M SPRINTS	REST	SETS

STAIRS RUNS, TAG & GO

||||||||||||||||||||||||||||||||||||||||||||

Start at the bottom of one flight of stairs (approximately 15–20 stairs). One of you should run up the stairs as fast as possible.

Once you reach the top of the stair, turn around and walk to the bottom – the other partner should go when you return to the bottom of the stairs.

THE NUMBERS

6-10	30 s	3
50M SPRINTS	REST	SETS

Gym training

|||||||||||||||||||||||||||||||||||||||||||||||||||||||||||||||||||||||

Strength training is at the core of our fitness programme. Its benefits are numerous, from increasing your bone density and improving your core muscles to helping you sleep better. Strength training builds muscle, which in turn helps raise your metabolism, meaning you will burn more calories (and therefore fat) each day than you would if you changed your diet alone.

Strength training isn't just a great workout for your body, it's also beneficial to your mind and well-being. Strength training has been shown to decrease stress levels, increase your endorphins and raise your self-confidence.

Combined with a healthy eating plan and HIIT, strength training will give you long-lasting improvements to your body. You will look good and feel great.

The following training routines are for beginning, intermediate and advanced levels of fitness.

We firmly believe that equipment and machines aren't just for people who have been gym-goers for years; quite the opposite in fact. If you're a beginner, don't be put off, ask for advice and then get stuck in.

Beginner workout

3-Day Training Week
Day 1: Lower body (legs & abs)
Day 2: Upper body
Day 3: Full body

Intermediate workout

4-Day Training Week
Day 1: Hamstrings, back & biceps
Day 2: Chest, triceps & shoulders
Day 3: Legs
Day 4: Chest, back & arms

Advanced workout

5-Day Training Week
Day 1: Legs & back
Day 2: Chest & shoulders
Day 3: Back & arms
Day 4: Legs & abs
Day 5: Full-body

TIP

If you have just joined a gym, or it's your first time using the equipment, don't be afraid to ask for advice and help from one of the resident trainers — that's what they are there for! And do seek advice on what weight to use; there is nothing worse than hurting yourself on the first day by using something that it is too heavy for you.

Beginner workout
day 1: lower body (legs & abs)

IIIIIIIIIIIIIIIIIIIIIIIIIIIIIIIIIIIIIIIIIIIIIIIIII

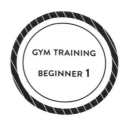

EXERCISE 1: QUAD EXTENSION

With your legs just within a shoulder width apart utilise the full range of motion you can comfortably achieve.

Squeeze through your quads at the peak and control the downward portion of the lift.

Keep your body still, with back and shoulders against the pads.

THE **NUMBERS**

10	60s	3
REPEATS	REST	SETS

EXERCISE 2: HAMSTRING CURLS

Push your back and shoulders against the pads, keeping the natural arch in your spine.

Ensure the base of your quads are against the pivot pad, legs shoulder width (or within) apart.

Squeeze through your hamstrings and draw your heels to your bum. Keep your body still, firmly grasping the handles.

THE **NUMBERS**

10	60s	3
REPEATS	REST	SETS

EXERCISE 3: LEG PRESS

Start with your back and shoulders against the pads and a neutral spine. Place your feet flat on the plate, shoulder width apart, pointing slightly outwards.

Push away from the plate until your legs are fully extended – avoid locking out your knees.

Control the return phase, utilising the range of motion that is comfortable.

THE **NUMBERS**

10	60s	3
REPEATS	REST	SETS
switch legs		

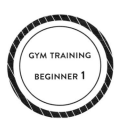

EXERCISE 4: GOBLET SQUATS

Set the feet just beyond shoulder width and grip a dumbbell as shown, pressed into the chest with you shoulders back.

Sink down as low as comfortably possible with the weight through your heels and back straight.

Drive upwards to standing, pressing evenly through the feet. Ensure you are balanced and repeat.

THE NUMBERS

15	60s	4
REPEATS	REST	SETS

EXERCISE 5: CRUNCHES SUPERSET TO RUSSIAN TWISTS

Lie flat on your back with the knees drawn towards you and feet flat on the floor.

Move the shoulders off the ground by flexing the spine, squeezing through the abs.

Slowly reverse the move, touch the head to the floor gently and repeat

//

Assume the top of a sit-up position but with your feet raised from the floor, elbows locked by your sides.

Grip a medicine ball/plate weight; twist from your core, move your torso and head in unity to one side, return to the centre then to the other side.

Avoid bouncing the weight and keep your legs pointing forwards.

THE NUMBERS

15/30	30s	4
REPEAT/S	REST	SETS

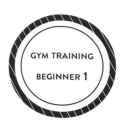

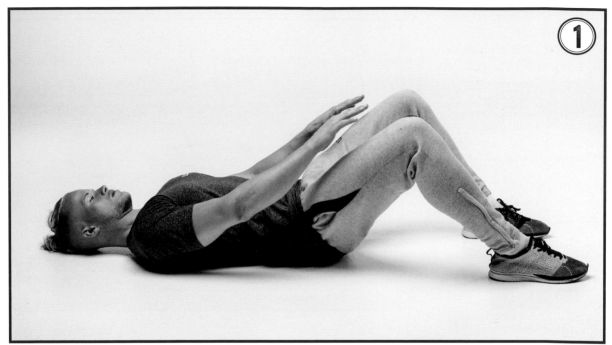

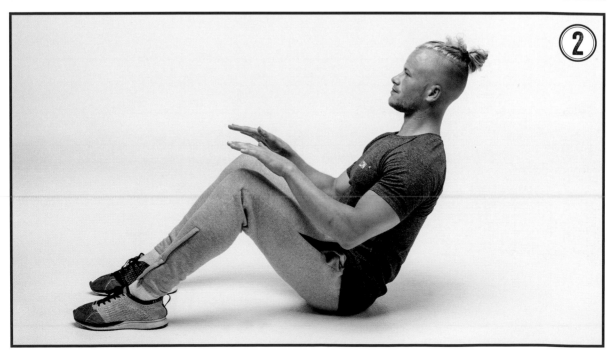

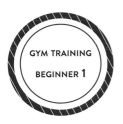

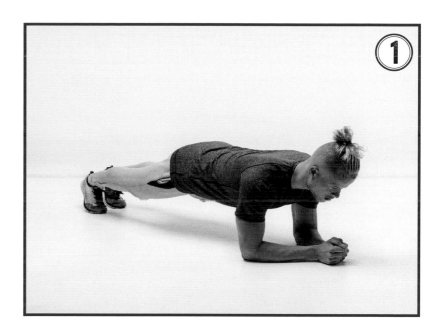

EXERCISE 6: PLANKS

Place your forearms flat on the floor with your elbows just within and directly below your shoulders.

Your body should be in a straight line from head to toe with your neck neutral.

Keep your core tight throughout and your breathing regular.

THE NUMBERS

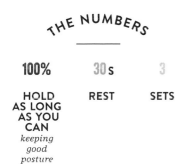

100%	30s	3
HOLD AS LONG AS YOU CAN *keeping good posture*	REST	SETS

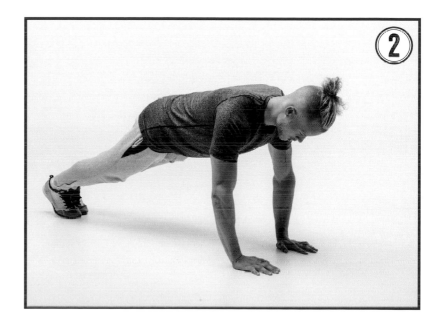

Beginner workout
day 2: upper body

||||||||||||||||||||||||||||||||||||||||||||||||||||||||||||||||

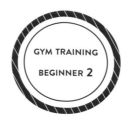

GYM TRAINING
BEGINNER 2

EXERCISE 1: LATERAL PULLDOWN
Take an overhand grip just outside your shoulder width.

Initiate the movement by contracting your scapula down and into place, then draw the elbows close past the sides until the bar touches just below your collarbone.

Maintain a small arch in the lower back and stretch the back at the peak by pushing upward slightly.

THE NUMBERS

10	60 s	3
REPEATS	**REST**	**SETS**
switch legs		

EXERCISE 2: SEATED CABLE ROW
Use an close-grip attachment with the hands facing each other.

Leaning back slightly with a slightly arched lower back, draw the attachment directly back into your belly button.

Squeeze through your back at the peak of the contraction. Feel a stretch through the back before returning to the start; repeat.

THE NUMBERS

10	60 s	3
REPEATS	**REST**	**SETS**
switch legs		

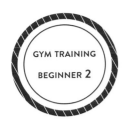

THE NUMBERS

10	60 s	3
REPEATS	**REST**	**SETS**

EXERCISE 3: DUMBBELL HAMMER SHOULDER PRESS

Take a dumbbell in each hand with a hammer grip– palms should face each other, and knuckles face upwards.

Start with the dumbbells slightly forward from your front delt, push directly upwards and squeeze through your shoulders.

Avoid locking your elbows, return in a controlled manner. Keep your elbows from flaring out.

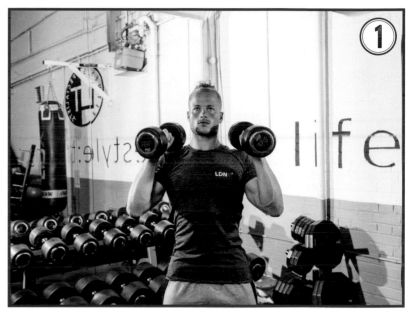

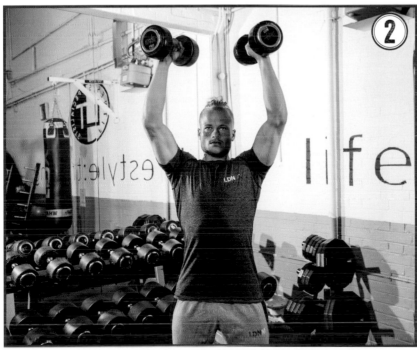

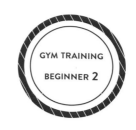
THE NUMBERS

10   **60**s   3

REPEATS   REST   SETS

EXERCISE 4: DUMBBELL LATERAL RAISES

Lean slightly forward. Lead with the elbow in these raises to prevent you swinging the weight up from your hands – dumbbells should be just above your shoulders at the peak of each rep.

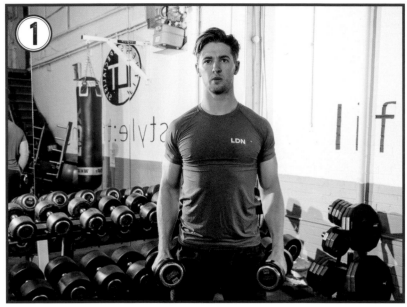

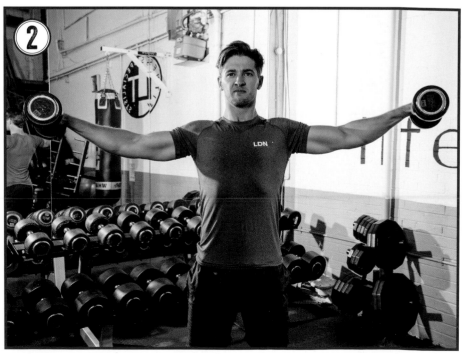

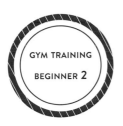

EXERCISE 5: DUMBBELL CHEST PRESS

Lay on your back on a flat bench, with the dumbbells above your chest and arms extended.

Move the dumbbells away from each other and downwards, until the elbow is level with the shoulders.

Press back up and together at the peak, before balancing and repeating.

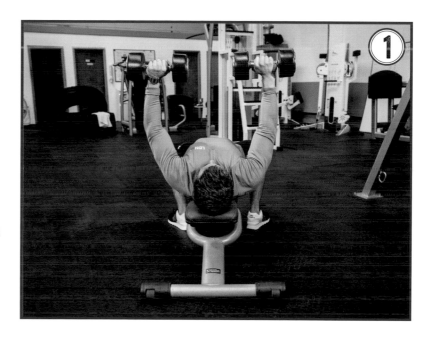

THE NUMBERS

10	60 s	3
REPEATS	REST	SETS

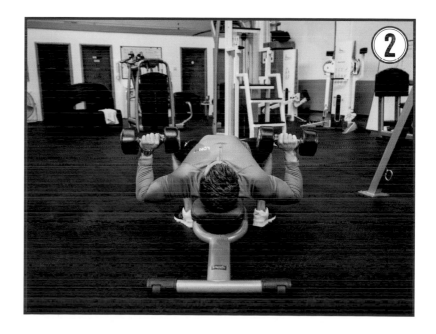

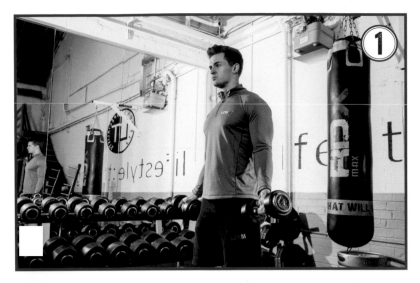

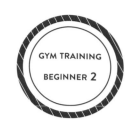

EXERCISE 6: BICEP CURLS

With your palms facing forwards, keep your elbows locked by your side.

Fully extend your arms at the bottom of the rep but keep the tension in your biceps.

Focus on controlled concentric/eccentric movements with a strong bicep contraction at the top of the rep.

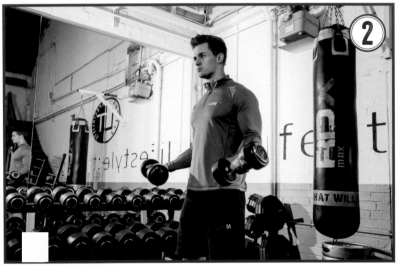

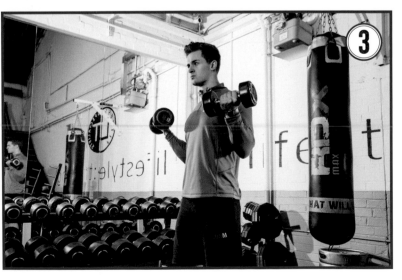

THE NUMBERS

10	60 s	3
REPEATS	**REST**	**SETS**
of biceps curls, followed immediately by tricep extensions		

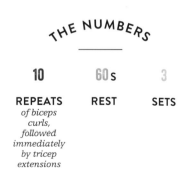

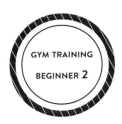

GYM TRAINING

BEGINNER **2**

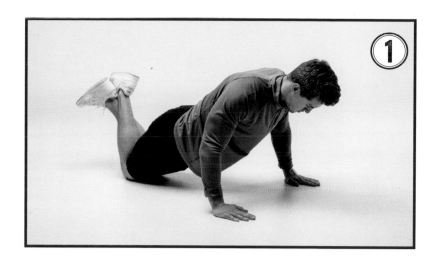

①

EXERCISE 7: PRESS UPS

Start with your hands slightly wider than your shoulders, arms fully extended.

Focus on keeping your body flat throughout the rep. Your elbows should stay close to your body, your chin almost touching the ground at the bottom of each rep. Push your body upwards.

Avoid locking out your elbows at the peak of the rep.

EASIER OPTION
perform on your knees

HARDER OPTION
full press up

THE NUMBERS

6-12	45 s	3
REPEATS	REST	SETS

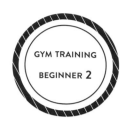

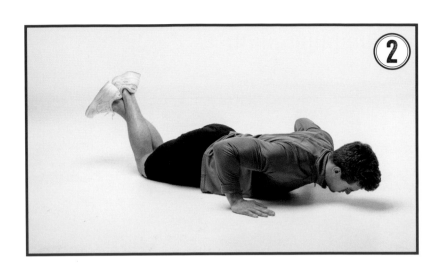

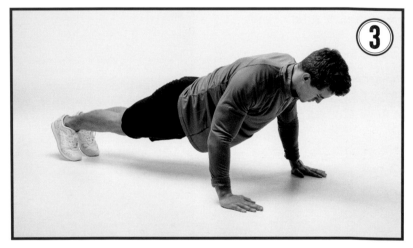

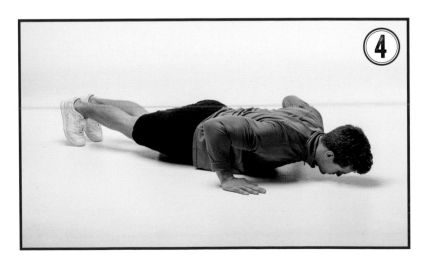

Beginner workout
day 3: full-body circuits

||||||||||||||||||||||||||||||||||||||||||||||||||||

Circuit 1

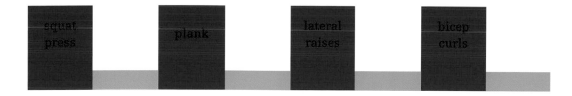

squat press

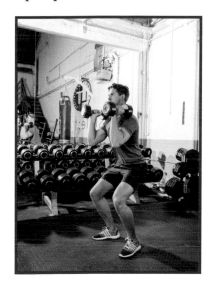
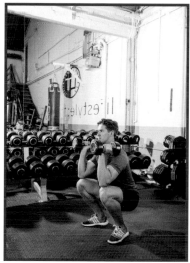
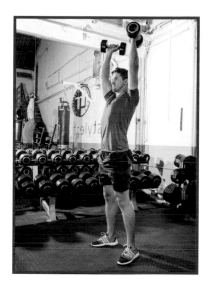

plank

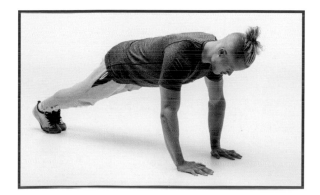

THE NUMBERS

20s
EACH EXERCISE

20s
REST
*between exercises
and between circuit*

3
SETS
each full circuit

2MN
REST
between each set

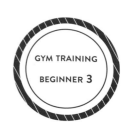

GYM TRAINING
BEGINNER **3**

lateral raises

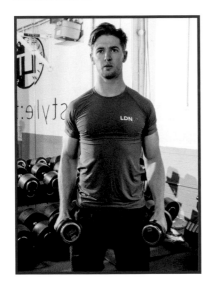
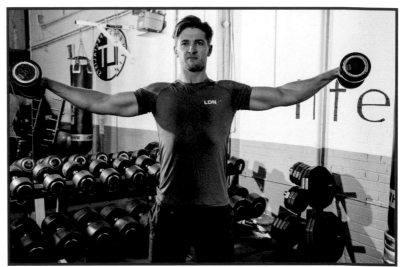

bicep curls

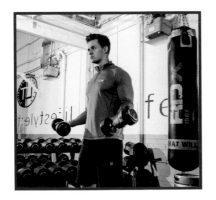
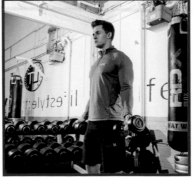
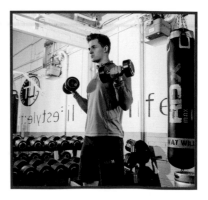

Circuit 2

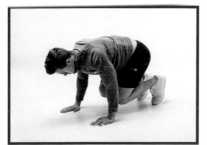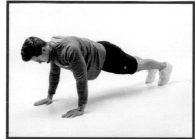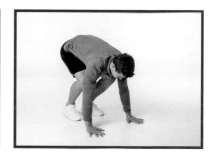

squat thrusts   tricep extensions   press ups   kettlebell swings

squat thrusts

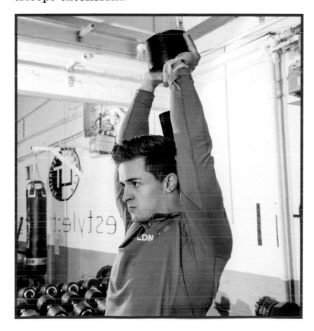

triceps extensions

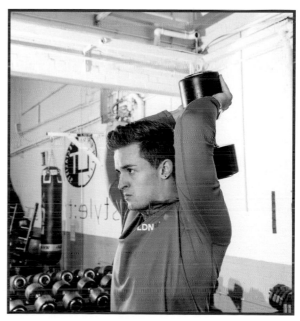

THE NUMBERS

20 s
EACH EXERCISE

20 s
REST
*between exercises
& between circuit*

3
SETS
each full circuit

2 MN
REST
between set

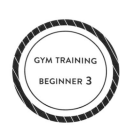
press ups

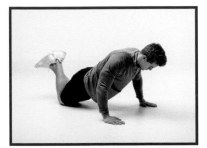
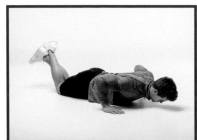
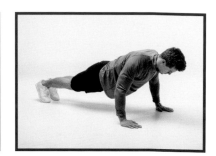

kettlebell swings

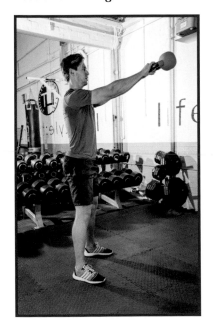
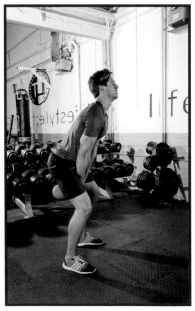
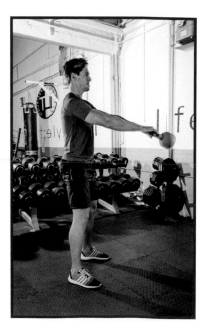

Intermediate workout
day 1: hamstrings, back, biceps
||||||||||||||||||||||||||||||||||||||||||||||||||||

EXERCISE 1: STIFF-LEG DEADLIFTS

Stand with feet 20–30cm apart with feet beneath the bar.

As you lower the weight bend your knees slightly, pivoting from the hips and keeping your back straight. When you feel a stretch in your hamstrings, this is the bottom of the rep.

Lift the bar by extending through your hips until standing upright. Pull shoulders back slightly if rounded. Extend knees at top if desired.

THE NUMBERS

10	75 s	3
REPEATS	REST	SETS

EXERCISE 2: HAMSTRING CURLS

Push your back and shoulders against the pads, keeping the natural arch in your spine.

Ensure the base of your quads are against the pivot pad, legs shoulder width (or within) apart.

Squeeze through your hamstrings and draw your heels to your bum. Keep your body still, firmly grasping the handles.

THE NUMBERS

8-12	45 s	7
REPEATS	REST	SETS

EXERCISE 3: LATERAL PULL DOWN

Take an overhand grip around 30cm outside your shoulder width. Initiate the movement with your lats rather than your biceps – sitting up straight, pull the bar down until it touches your upper chest.

THE NUMBERS

8-10	75 s	4
REPEATS	REST	SETS

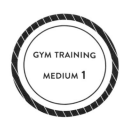

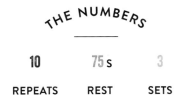

THE NUMBERS

10	75 s	3
REPEATS	REST	SETS

EXERCISE 4: SINGLE-ARM DUMBBELL ROW

Select a flat bench and dumbbell, and then place one leg on the bench and brace with your arm.

Keeping your back flat and body still, draw your elbow up and backwards – drawing the dumbbell towards your hip.

Squeeze your back before lowering until you feel a stretch through your back and repeat.

THE NUMBERS

10	75 s	3
REPEATS	REST	SETS

EXERCISE 5: STRAIGHT-ARM PULL DOWN

Using the rope attachment, push the weight downwards before drawing it towards your hips and squeezing your shoulders back.

Assume a 45-degree angle of your body to the ground throughout, with your knees slightly bent and body still.

Squeeze your back at the base, and feel a stretch at the peak.

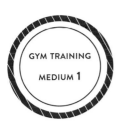

GYM TRAINING

MEDIUM 1

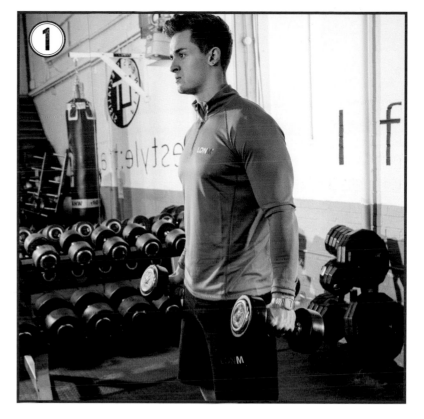

EXERCISE 6: DUMBBELL HAMMER CURLS

Keep elbows in tight beside your body. At the peak of the rep there should be a 45-degree angle between your upper arm and forearm, squeezing through the bicep.

THE NUMBERS

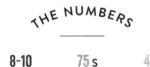

8-10	75 s	4
REPEATS	REST	SETS
each sides, alternating		

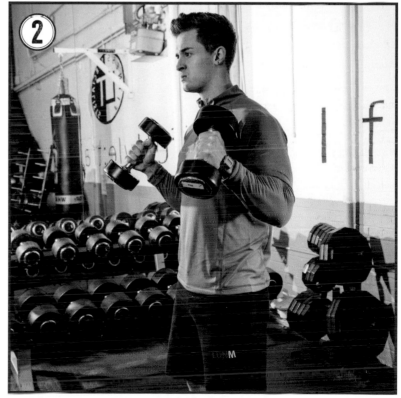

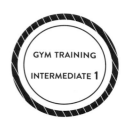
EXERCISE 7: ZOTTMAN CURLS

Stand tall with good posture and your palms facing forwards.

Curl to the peak of the rep by flexing your elbows, and then rotate the dumbbells so your palms face away from your body.

Lower the dumbbells slowly, and when you reach the base turn the dumbbells again so that your palms face away, and repeat.

THE NUMBERS

10	75 s	3
RE-PEATS*	REST	SETS

* Repeat of biceps curls, followed immediately by tricep extensions

EXERCISE 8: REVERSE BARBELL CURLS

Take an overhand grip of the bar with your hands shoulder width apart, keeping your elbows close by your sides.

Fully extend your elbows at the bottom of the rep.

Focus on a strong upward and controlled downward movement, with a strong contraction through your biceps at the top of the rep.

THE NUMBERS

12	75 s	3
REPEATS	REST	SETS

Intermediate workout
day 2: chest, triceps & shoulders
||||||||||||||||||||||||||||||||||||||||||||||||||||||

EXERCISE 1: BENCH PRESS

Take a comfortable, slightly wider than shoulder width, grip on the bar. Un-rack the bar safely to the starting position before lowering until it touches your nipples/sternum.

Breathe in and push directly upwards – through your chest rather than shoulders.

Avoid locking out your elbows at the peak of one movement.

THE NUMBERS

8-10	75 s	4
REPEATS	REST	SETS

EXERCISE 2: ARNOLD PRESS

Select a weights bench 1–2 notches off vertical and sit with good posture, with your palms facing your chest.

Push the dumbbells upwards, and draw your elbows outwards throughout so that your palms face forwards at the peak.

Control the descent and reverse the movement before repeating.

THE NUMBERS

8	75 s	4
REPEATS	REST	SETS

EXERCISE 3: INCLINE DUMBBELL FLYES

Set the bench to a 15–30 degree incline. Start with your arms extended, dumbbells above your chest with palms facing each other.

Lead the movement from your hands, while keeping your elbows in line with your shoulders.

Go as low as comfortably possible while maintaining form. Control the upwards phase by contracting your chest.

THE NUMBERS

10	75 s	3
REPEATS	REST	SETS
each sides		

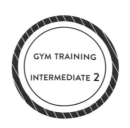
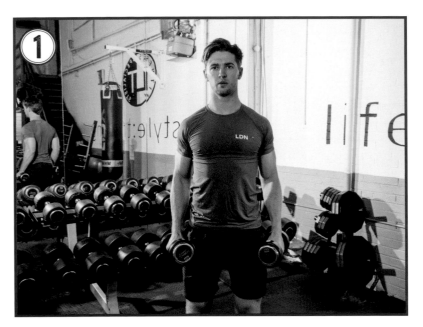

EXERCISE 4: DUMBBELL LATERAL RAISES

Lean slightly forwards. Lead with the elbow in these raises to prevent you swinging the weight up from your hands – dumbbells should be just above your shoulders at the peak of each rep.

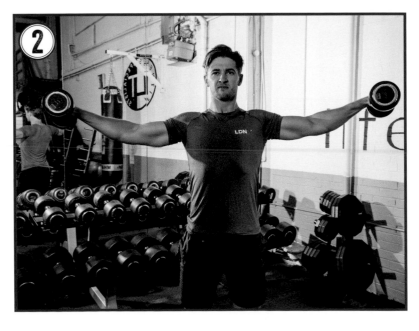

THE NUMBERS

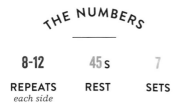

8-12	45 s	7
REPEATS *each side*	**REST**	**SETS**

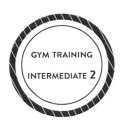

THE NUMBERS

10	75 s	3
REPEATS *each sides*	**REST**	**SETS**

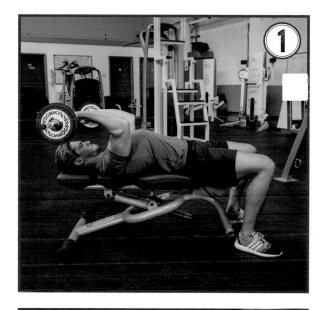

EXERCISE 5: EZ BAR SKULL CRUSHERS

Keep your elbows directly above your shoulders throughout the rep – do not allow them to bow outwards or move down towards your hips.

Start with straight arms, flexing at the elbows – stop the bar at your hairline at the base of each repetition.

Squeeze through your triceps on the upward phase until the elbows extend fully.

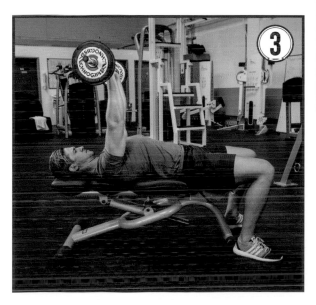

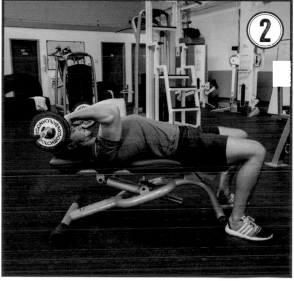

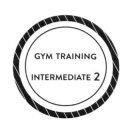

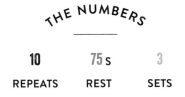

8-10   **75** s   *4*

REPEATS   **REST**   **SETS**
each side,
alternating

EXERCISE 6: TRICEP PULL DOWNS

Use a flat bar attachment on a high cable. Stand tall and keep your elbows in throughout.

Start with a 90-degree angle at your elbows, draw the attachment down towards your crotch and fully extend your triceps at the peak of the movement.

Control the return to the start position and repeat.

THE NUMBERS

10   **75** s   *3*

REPEATS   **REST**   **SETS**

EXERCISE 7: TRICEP KICKBACKS

Select a pair of dumbbells. Take up a shoulder-width stance and get your body as parallel to the floor as possible, while keeping the back flat.

Keep your elbows high, and upper arms parallel to the ground, before extending and flexing your elbows simultaneously.

Control the speed throughout and maintain your posture.

Intermediate workout
day 3: legs & abs

||||||||||||||||||||||||||||||||||||||||||||||||||||||

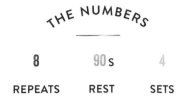

THE NUMBERS

8	90s	4
REPEATS	REST	SETS

EXERCISE 1: STIFF-LEG BARBELL DEADLIFTS

Stand with feet 20–30cm apart with feet beneath the bar.

As you lower the weight bend your knees slightly, pivoting from the hips and keeping your back straight.

When you feel a stretch in your hamstrings, this is the bottom of the rep. Lift the bar by extending through the hips until standing upright. Pull your shoulders back slightly if rounded.

Extend your knees at the top if desired.

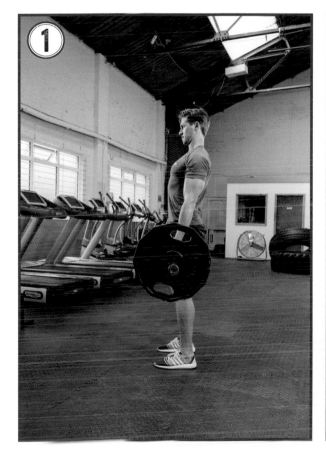

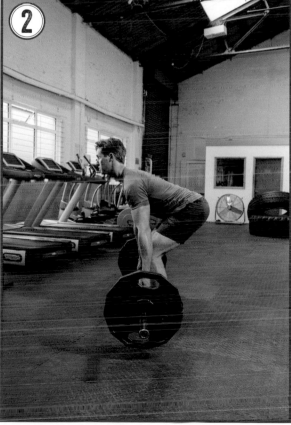

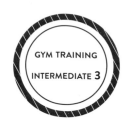

THE NUMBERS
————

10-12	90s	4
REPEATS	REST	SETS
heavy		

EXERCISE 2: QUAD EXTENSION

With your legs just within or shoulder width apart, utilise the full range of motion you can comfortably achieve.

Squeeze through your quads at the peak, and control the downward portion of the lift.

Keep your body still, and back and shoulders against the pads.

EXERCISE 3: BARBELL SQUATS

Place your feet shoulder width apart, with the bar across your traps, grip the bar outside of shoulder width, elbows in.

Break from your hips; your bum should move back and down, weight through your heels.

Sink to just below parallel, maintaining a strong core and straight spine – powerfully drive up to standing. Keep looking forwards throughout.

THE NUMBERS
————

8	90s	4
REPEATS	REST	SETS
each sides		

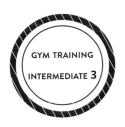

EXERCISE 4: HAMSTRING CURLS

Push your back and shoulders against the pads, keeping the natural arch in your spine.

Ensure that the base of your quads are against the pivot pad, legs shoulder width (or within) apart.

Squeeze through your hamstrings and draw your heels to your bum. Keep your body still, firmly grasping the handles.

THE NUMBERS

10-12	75 s	4
REPEATS *heavy*	REST	SETS

EXERCISE 5: BULGARIAN SPLIT SQUATS
(see visual opposite)

Similar stance to static lunges, except rear foot should be on a bench/box around knee height.

Squat down until front leg is parallel to the ground, keeping tension through glutes and thigh.

THE NUMBERS

10	75 s	3
REPEATS *each leg*	REST	SETS

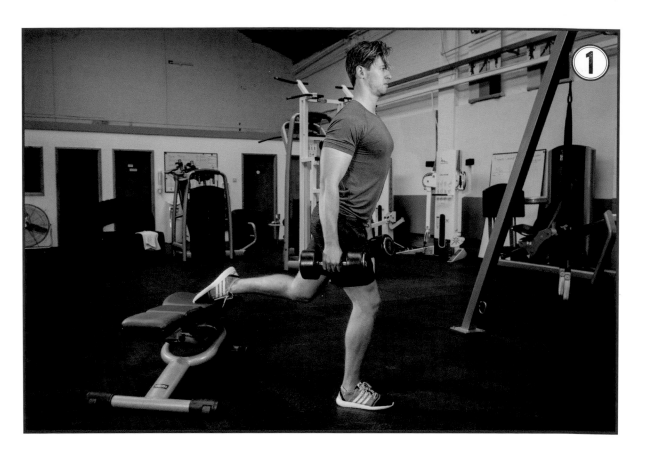

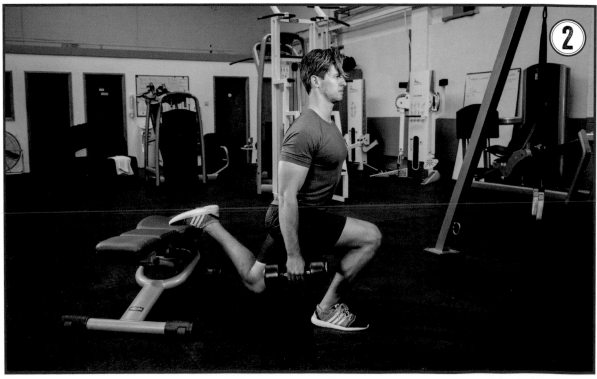

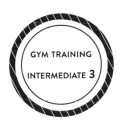

EXERCISE 6: FEET RAISED WEIGHTED CRUNCHES

Assume your starting crunch position, with a weight of your choice to hand.

Lift your legs into the 90-degree table-top position. Pick up the weight and, keeping your arms straight, try and push the weight up to the ceiling, looking up as you go.

Your back should lift off the floor as you go up; lower your back gently to the floor and repeat the movement.

THE NUMBERS

10-12	45 s	3
REPEATS	REST	SETS

EXERCISE 7: LYING LEG RAISES

(see visual opposite)

Lie flat on a mat with your arms by your side, or beneath the bum if this is more comfortable.

Lift your feet upwards until the feet are directly above the hips, keeping the legs straight.

In a controlled manner return to the starting position, but do not allow your feet to touch the mat. Repeat.

THE NUMBERS

15	30 s	4
REPEATS	REST	SETS

EXERCISE 8: RUSSIAN TWISTS

Assume the top of a sit-up position but with your feet raised from the floor, elbows locked by your sides.

Grip a medicine ball/plate weight; twist from your core, move your torso and head in unison to one side, return to the centre, then to the other side.

Avoid bouncing the weight and keep your legs pointing forwards.

THE NUMBERS

30	30 s	4
REPEATS	REST	SETS

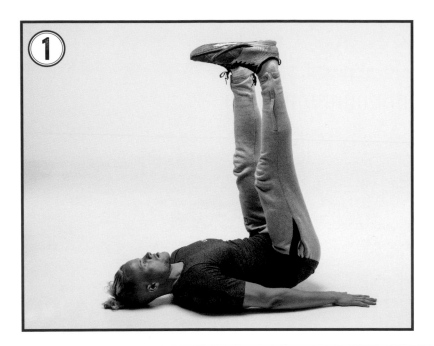

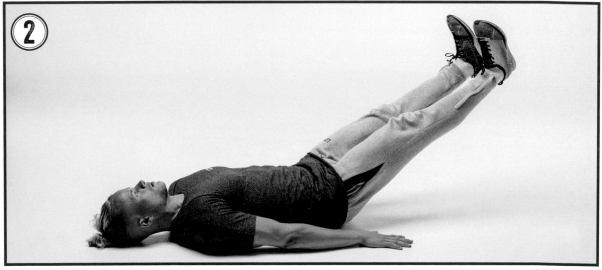

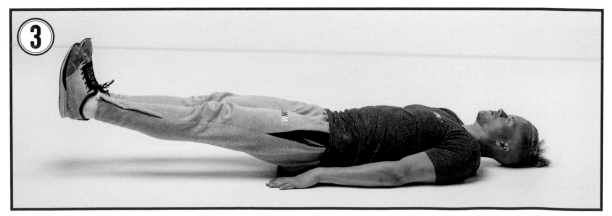

Intermediate workout
day 4: chest, back & arms
|||||||||||||||||||||||||||||||||||||||||||||||||||||||||

EXERCISE 1: BENT OVER ROW
With soft knees and your torso leant forwards keep the back flat throughout.

Take a shoulder width overhand grip and draw the bar into your belly button, keeping your elbows close to your ribs.

Slowly lower to the base of the rep, feeling a stretch through the back before repeating.

THE NUMBERS

10	60s	4
REPEATS	REST	SETS
heavy		

EXERCISE 2: DECLINE BENCH PRESS
Opt for a 15–30-degree declined bench and grip the bar just outside shoulder width.

Lower the bar slowly until it touches the lower chest, before driving the bar away from you until your elbows are almost fully extended.

Ensure you are balanced and then repeat the move.

THE NUMBERS

10	60s	4
REPEATS	REST	SETS

EXERCISE 3: LATERAL PULL DOWN
Take an overhand grip just outside of your shoulder width.

Initiate the movement by contracting your scapula down and into place, then draw the elbows close past the side, until the bar touches just below your collarbone.

Maintain a small arch in your lower back, and stretch your back at the peak by pushing upward slightly.

THE NUMBERS

12	60s	3
REPEATS	REST	SETS
each leg		

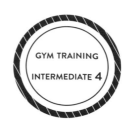

THE NUMBERS

12	60 s	3
REPEATS	REST	SETS

EXERCISE 4: INCLINE DUMBBELL PRESS
Set a bench to a 15–30 degree incline.

Press the dumbbells upwards above your chest, stopping just before your elbows fully straighten.

Lower the dumbbells until they are level with your chest and in line with your nipples, before driving them back upwards.

THE NUMBERS

10	60 s	5
REPEATS	REST	SETS

EXERCISE 5: BARBELL CURLS
Stand tall, gripping the bar at shoulder width with your palms facing away from you and elbows straight.

Keep your elbow still and close to your sides, before flexing the elbows by contracting your biceps.

Lower the barbell slowly, until your elbows straighten, before repeating the move.

THE NUMBERS

10	60 s	5
REPEATS	REST	SETS

EXERCISE 6: TRICEP ROPE PULL DOWNS
Keep your elbows by your side, extend your triceps fully – at the bottom of the rep, twist your hands so the bottom of them are pointing outwards, while maintaining tension through your triceps.

Advanced workout
day 1: legs & back

||||||||||||||||||||||||||||||||||||||||||||||||||||||||

EXERCISE 1: DEADLIFTS

With your feet flat beneath the bar, squat down and grasp the bar at shoulder width with an overhand or mixed grip.

Lift the bar by extending your hips and knees to full extension simultaneously. Pull your shoulders back at the top and push your chest out.

Reset starting position between each rep.

THE NUMBERS

5	90 s	5
REPEATS	REST	SETS

EXERCISE 2: LATERAL PULL DOWN

Take an overhand grip just outside of your shoulder width.

Initiate the movement by contracting your scapula down and into place, then draw your elbows close to your ribs until the bar touches just below your collarbone.

Maintain a small arch in your lower back, and stretch your back at the peak by pushing upward slightly.

THE NUMBERS

12	90 s	4
REPEATS	REST	SETS

EXERCISE 3: LEG PRESS

Start with your back and shoulders against the pads and a neutral spine. Place your feet flat on the plate, shoulder width apart, pointing slightly outwards.

Push away from the plate until your legs are fully extended – avoid locking out your knees.

Control the return phase, utilising the range of motion that is comfortable.

THE NUMBERS

15	90 s	4
REPEATS	REST	SETS

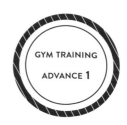

THE NUMBERS

15	90 s	3
REPEATS	REST	SETS

EXERCISE 4: SEATED CABLE ROW

Use a close grip attachment with your hands facing each other.

Leaning back slightly with a slightly arched lower back, draw the attachment directly back into your belly button.

Squeeze through your back at the peak of the contraction. Feel a stretch through the back before returning to the start; repeat.

THE NUMBERS

15	60 s	3
REPEATS	REST	SETS

EXERCISE 5: HAMSTRING CURLS

Push your back and shoulders against the pads, keeping the natural arch in your spine.

Ensure the base of your quads are against the pivot pad, legs shoulder width (or within) apart.

Squeeze through your hamstrings and draw your heels to your bum. Keep your body still, firmly grasping the handles.

THE NUMBERS

12	30 s	7
REPEATS	REST	SETS

EXERCISE 6: DUMBBELL SHRUGS

Place your feet shoulder width apart, dumbbells by your side, palms facing inwards and with your shoulders pulled back.

Shrug your shoulders upwards, contracting your trapezius; pause for a second before controlling the dumbbells during the eccentric and stretching the traps at the base of each rep.

Keep your head and neck neutral.

Advanced workout
day 2: chest & shoulders

||||||||||||||||||||||||||||||||||||||||||||||||||||||||||||

EXERCISE 1: BENCH PRESS

Take a comfortable, slightly wider than shoulder width, grip on the bar. Un-rack the bar safely to the starting position before lowering until it touches your nipples/sternum.

Breathe in and push directly upwards – through your chest rather than shoulders.

Avoid locking out your elbows at the peak of the movement.

THE NUMBERS

8	90 s	4
REPEATS	REST	SETS

EXERCISE 2: STANDING DUMBBELL SHOULDER PRESS

Set your feet at shoulder width, with soft knees, squeezing the glutes and maintaining good posture. Start with the dumbbells just outside shoulder width.

Drive the dumbbells upwards and then smoothly inward as you squeeze your shoulder at the peak.

Lower slowly to the start position and then repeat. Avoid locking out the knees or elbows.

THE NUMBERS

8	90 s	4
REPEATS	REST	SETS

EXERCISE 3: INCLINE DUMBBELL PRESS

Set a bench to a 15–30 degree incline.

Press the dumbbells upwards above the chest, stopping just before the elbows fully straighten.

Lower the dumbbells until they are level with the chest and in line with the nipples, before driving them back upwards.

THE NUMBERS

10	75 s	3
REPEATS	REST	SETS

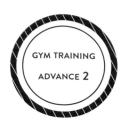

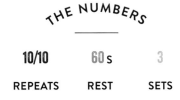

THE NUMBERS

10/10
REPEATS

75 s
REST

3
SETS

EXERCISE 4: UPRIGHT ROWS

Stand tall and grip the barbell at shoulder width with your palms facing you, and lean your torso forwards slightly with your back flat.

Draw your elbows upwards until they are in line with your ears and squeeze your shoulders back.

Lower slowly until your elbows straighten, and then repeat.

THE NUMBERS

10/10
REPEATS

60 s
REST

3
SETS

EXERCISE 5: PLATE SQUEEZE RAISES SUPERSET TO FRONT PLATE RAISE

Select a weight plate and squeeze it between the palms of your hands to prevent it falling, keeping a constant and small bend at your elbows.

Maintain this pressure and raise the plate from in front of your crotch to chest height.

Slowly lower back to the base and repeat (maintaining good posture throughout).

//

Stand up straight; with your feet shoulder width apart, neutral spine.

Hold the plate at 3 and 9 o'clock and with straight arms, raise the plate until your hands are in-line with your shoulders.

Pause for a second before controlling the lowering phase.

Advanced workout
day 3: back & arms

||||||||||||||||||||||||||||||||||||||||||||||||||||||||||||

EXERCISE 1: LATERAL PULL DOWN

Take an overhand grip just outside of your shoulder width.

Initiate the movement by contracting your scapula down and into place, then draw the elbows close past the sides until the bar touches just below your collarbone.

Maintain a small arch in your lower back, and stretch your back at the peak by pushing upward slightly.

THE NUMBERS

15	75 s	4
REPEATS	REST	SETS

EXERCISE 2: SEATED CABLE ROWS

Use a close grip attachment with your hands facing each other.

Leaning back slightly with a slightly arched lower back, draw the attachment directly back into your belly button.

Squeeze through your back at the peak of the contraction. Feel a stretch through your back before returning to the start; repeat.

THE NUMBERS

15	75 s	4
REPEATS	REST	SETS

EXERCISE 3: STRAIGHT-ARM PULL DOWNS

Select a flat bar or rope attachment.

Lean the torso forwards to a 45-degree angle with the floor, arms extended overhead and your back flat.

Push your hands down and then draw them into your waist. Keep your arms straight throughout, reverse the arced motion and repeat.

THE NUMBERS

20	60 s	3
REPEATS	REST	SETS

EXERCISE 4: DUMBBELL SHRUGS

Place your feet shoulder width apart, dumbbells by your side, palms facing inwards and with your shoulders pulled back.

Shrug your shoulders upwards, contracting your trapezius; pause for a second before controlling the dumbbells during the eccentric and stretching the traps at the base of each rep.

Keep your head and neck neutral.

THE NUMBERS

12	75 s	4
REPEATS	REST	SETS

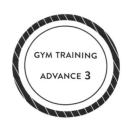

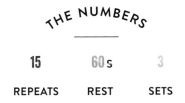

THE NUMBERS

10/10	75 s	4
REPEATS	REST	SETS

EXERCISE 5: BARBELL CURLS SUPERSET TO SKULL CRUSHERS

Stand tall, gripping the bar at shoulder width with your palms facing away from you and elbows straight.

Keep your elbow still and close to your sides, before flexing the elbows by contracting the biceps.

Lower the barbell slowly, until your elbows straighten, before repeating the move.

//

Keep your elbows directly above your shoulders throughout the rep – do not allow them to bow outwards or move down towards your hips.

Start with straight arms, flexing at the elbows – stop the bar at your hairline at the base of each repetition.

Squeeze through your triceps on the upward phase until your elbows extend fully.

THE NUMBERS

15	60 s	3
REPEATS	REST	SETS

EXERCISE 6: TRICEP KICKBACKS

Select a pair of dumbbells at shoulder-width stance and get your body as parallel to the floor as possible, while keeping the back flat.

Keep the elbows high and upper arms parallel to the ground, before extending and flexing your elbows simultaneously.

Control the speed throughout and maintain your posture.

Advanced workout
day 4: legs & abs

‖‖‖

EXERCISE 1: BARBELL SQUATS

Place your feet shoulder width apart, with the bar across your traps, grip the bar outside shoulder width, elbows in.

Break from your hips; your bum should move back and down, weight through your heels.

Sink to just below parallel, maintaining a strong core and straight spine – powerfully drive up to standing. Keep looking forwards throughout.

THE NUMBERS

15	75 s	4
REPEATS	REST	SETS

EXERCISE 2: LEG PRESS

Start with your back and shoulders against the pads and a neutral spine. Place your feet flat on the plate, shoulder width apart, pointing slightly outwards.

Push away from the plate until your legs are fully extended – avoid locking out your knees.

Control the return phase, utilising the range of motion that is comfortable.

THE NUMBERS

15	75 s	4
REPEATS	REST	SETS

EXERCISE 3: STIFF-LEG DEADLIFTS

Stand with feet 20–30cm apart with feet beneath the bar.

As you lower the weight bend your knees slightly, pivoting from the hips and keep your back straight. When you feel a stretch in your hamstrings, this is the bottom of the rep.

Lift bar by extending through your hips until standing upright. Pull shoulders back slightly if rounded.

Extend knees at top if desired.

THE NUMBERS

20	60 s	3
REPEATS	REST	SETS

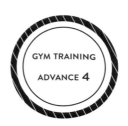

THE NUMBERS

12	75 s	4
REPEATS	REST	SETS

EXERCISE 4: HAMSTRING CURLS

Push your back and shoulders against the pads, keeping the natural arch in your spine.

Ensure the base of your quads are against the pivot pad, legs shoulder width (or within) apart.

Squeeze through your hamstrings and draw your heels to your bum. Keep your body still, firmly grasping the handles.

THE NUMBERS

10/10	75 s	4
REPEATS	REST	SETS

EXERCISE 5: QUAD EXTENSION

With your legs just within or shoulder width apart utilise the full range of motion you can comfortably achieve.

Squeeze through your quads at the peak and control the downward portion of the lift.

Keep your body still, and back and shoulders against the pads.

THE NUMBERS

15	60 s	3
REPEATS	REST	SETS

EXERCISE 6: CALF EXTENSIONS

Your back and shoulders should be pushed against the pads, preserving a natural arch in your back.

Place the balls of your feet on the plate, so that your heels are over the edge, and extend your legs.

Keep your legs straight; push through the ball of your foot to fully extend your calfs, contracting strongly at the peak.

Advanced workout
day 5: full body

||||||||||||||||||||||||||||||||||||||||||||||||||||||||||||

EXERCISE 1: DEADLIFTS

With your feet flat beneath the bar, squat down and grasp the bar at shoulder width with an over-hand or mixed grip.

Lift the bar by extending your hips and knees to full extension simultaneously. Pull your shoulders back at the top and push your chest out.

Reset starting position between each rep.

THE NUMBERS

8	90 s	4
REPEATS	REST	SETS

EXERCISE 2: DUMBELL CHEST PRESS

Keep the dumbbells in line with your nose throughout the movement – ensuring elbows stop slightly below your shoulders at the base of each repetition. Your back should be in a 'natural straight position', not overly arched or completely straight.

THE NUMBERS

10	75 s	4
REPEATS	REST	SETS

EXERCISE 3: LATERAL PULL DOWN

Take an overhand grip just outside at your shoulder width.

Initiate the movement by contracting your scapula down and into place, then draw your elbows close past the side until the bar touches just below your collarbone.

Maintain a small arch in your lower back and stretch the back at the peak by pushing upward slightly.

THE NUMBERS

12	75 s	4
REPEATS	REST	SETS

EXERCISE 4: MILITARY PRESS

Place your feet slightly wider than shoulder width apart (staggered if preferred).

Grip the bar, hands shoulder width apart, or slightly wider; start with it touching your chest just below your collarbone.

Press upwards, stopping just before full extension of your elbows. Control the return phase.

THE NUMBERS

10	75 s	4
REPEATS	REST	SETS

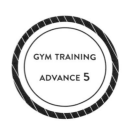

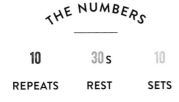

10/12	75 s	4
REPEATS	REST	SETS

EXERCISE 5:
SKULL CRUSHERS SUPERSET TO HAMMER CURLS

Keep your elbows directly above your shoulders throughout the rep – do not allow them to bow outwards or move down towards your hips.

Start with straight arms, flexing at the elbows – stop the bar at your hairline at the base of each repetition.

Squeeze through your triceps on the upward phase until the elbows extend fully.

//

Keep elbows in tight beside your body. At the peak of the rep there should be a 45-degree angle between your upper arm and forearm, squeezing through the bicep.

THE NUMBERS

10	30 s	10
REPEATS	REST	SETS

EXERCISE 6: BURPEES

Assume a press-up position and jump both feet in, tucking your knees under your torso, before jumping vertically and extending your body.

Land softly and place your hands in the same position, before jumping your feet back out to a start position.

Repeat at a fast pace.

Stretches

||||||||||||||||||||||||||||||||||||||||||||||||||

Stretching before and after a workout improves flexibility and helps to avoid injury. But you also run the risk of injury if you stretch when your body is cold, so do a couple of minutes of light cardio first; 50 star jumps are just about right to get your muscles warm.

LOWER BODY
||||||||||||||||||||||||||||||||||||||||||||||

Do them at home after leg days and sports such as football, tennis and swimming, and try to complete them at least once a day – try doing them in front of the TV or when waiting for the kettle to boil.

Incorporate them into your lifting routine and see if your recovery, range of motion (squat depth and form especially) and conditioning improves.

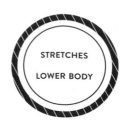

STRETCHES

LOWER BODY

HAMSTRING STRETCH

1 / From a seated position on the floor, extend one leg out directly in front of you and rest it flat on the floor.

2 / Reach forwards towards your foot with both hands until a mildly uncomfortable stretch is felt down the back of the extended leg.

3 / Hold for 20–30 seconds.

4 / Relax and sit up for 5 seconds, before exhaling and pushing slightly further in the same stretch position, and holding this increased stretch for a further 10 seconds.

5 / Repeat the process for the opposite leg.

GLUTE STRETCH

1 / Lie flat on the floor and bring one knee up towards your chest, then pull your heel towards the shoulder on the opposite side of your body.

2 / Bring the knee of the opposite leg up and apply pressure to the ankle until you feel a stretch in the glute area of the adducted leg.

3 / You may wish to support the leg, applying the stretching force with your arms to increase the stretch.

4 / Hold the stretch for 30 seconds, increasing the stretch slightly for the duration.

5 / Repeat the stretch on the other side.

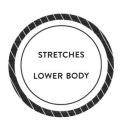

GROIN STRETCH

1 / Seated on the floor, bring the soles of your feet together so they touch.

2 / Now with both hands pull your feet towards you until your heels are a couple of inches from your body.

3 / With your hands on your feet apply pressure to the inside of your knees with your elbows, pushing your knees outwards and downwards towards the floor until a stretch is felt in your groin.

4 / Hold for 25–30 seconds.

HIP FLEXOR STRETCH

1 / Take an extended lunge position, ensuring your rear knee is behind your body, not directly below it.

2 / Keeping your body upright, lean your legs forwards to increase the stretch on the hip flexor of your rear leg.

3 / To increase the stretch further lean your torso backwards and twist away from the rear leg – you may pull on a stationary object for support and/or an increased stretch.

4 / Hold this stretch for 30–40 seconds before switching legs.

QUAD STRETCH

1 / This stretch can be performed kneeling or standing.

2 / Holding your ankle, pull it upwards towards your bum, while keeping your knees together and hips level and neutral, and your body straight and upright – you should feel a stretch throughout the quad.

3 / To increase the stretch lean your torso backwards.

4 / Switch to the other leg.

CALF STRETCH

1 / From a press-up position, raise your bum slightly and place one leg across the back of the other.

2 / Straighten the working leg and drop your heel towards the floor to stretch your calf.

3 / Lower your hips to increase the stretch.

4 / Repeat on the other leg.

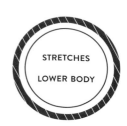

ERECTOR SPINE STRETCH

1 / Lying flat on your back, raise your knees until there is a rough right angle at your hip and knees.

2 / Holding just below your knees, pull them into your chest so that a stretch is felt in your lower back and hip region.

3 / Hold for 5 seconds before releasing the stretch and flattening your back for 2–3 seconds.

4 / Repeat this process 5 times.

ABDOMINAL STRETCH

1 / From a press-up position, keep your pelvis on the floor while you straighten your arms and look upwards.

2 / Walk your hands towards your body to increase the stretch, and away to lessen it. Hold the stretch for 20–30 seconds.

HIP/OBLIQUE STRETCH

1 / In a standing position with your feet just less than a shoulder width apart, raise your arms upwards and clasp your hands together above your head.

2 / Lean to one side and don't allow your hips or shoulders to twist, you should feel a stretch through your outer hip and oblique region on the opposite side to the direction that you are leaning.

3 / Repeat on the other side.

Repeat this routine twice through, and aim to increase the intensity of the stretches on the second round to a safe degree.

UPPER BODY

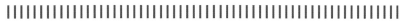

Make sure that your body isn't cold when you perform these stretches. Take a shower first or do some light cardio. This is a great stretching routine to incorporate into your training regimen to allow for improved performance, reduced likelihood of injury and to generally improve overall conditioning for sport, lifting and day-to-day activities.

If you are aware of any injury or condition that a progressive stretching routine may aggravate, please seek medical advice before performing the below.

STRETCHING CAT

1 / Assume a four-point crawl position.

2 / Arch your back by pushing your abdomen towards the ground and raise your head up/backwards.

3 / Do this until you feel a stretch through the abdominal muscles.

If this aggravates a back/stomach injury please avoid and/or proceed with caution.

PRONE ABDOMINAL STRETCH

1 / Assume the top of a press-up position and then allow your legs to lie flat on the ground.

2 / Walk your hands back slowly towards your body until you feel a stretch through your abs.

3 / Keep your upper thighs/hips on the ground throughout.

If this aggravates a back/stomach injury please avoid and/or proceed with caution.

ANGRY CAT

1 / Assume a four-point crawl position and draw your belly button in to your spine.

2 / Round your back upwards, with your head looking at the floor below your chest, until you feel a stretch across your back.

3 / Walk your hands in towards your legs to increase the stretch.

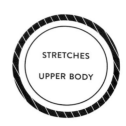
STANDING BACK STRETCH

1 / From a standing position, let your torso hang forwards by bending at the hip and allowing your spine/back to flex.

2 / Keep your legs straight and allow your spine/back to flex until a stretch is felt through your back, hips and glutes/ hamstrings.

KNEELING BACK STRETCH

1 / Assume a four-point crawl position.

2 / Take your right hand and draw it under your body until the outside of your right elbow is touching your left hand/wrist.

3 / Place your left hand on the top of the right and sit your bum down towards the feet until you feel a stretch through the right side and base of your back.

4 / Repeat on the other side.

TIP

Don't underestimate the importance of stretching: stretching improves flexibility, blood flow and nutrient supply to your muscles, as well as providing a bit of calm. Trust us – your bodies will thank you later.

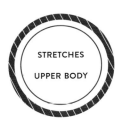

SCAPULA/DELT STRETCH (A)

1 / Assume a standing position and draw your right arm across your body so it is horizontal. Place your left palm at the base of your elbow.

2 / Keep your right arm straight while retracting your left shoulder (pulling your right arm towards your chest) to increase the stretch.

3 / Keep your right palm facing behind your body throughout.

4 / Repeat on the other side.

SCAPULA/DELT STRETCH (B)

1 / Assume a standing position and draw your right arm across your body so it is horizontal. Place your left palm at the base of your elbow.

2 / Keep your right arm straight while retracting your left shoulder (pulling your right arm towards your chest) to increase the stretch.

3 / Keep your right palm facing away from your body, with your thumb down, throughout the stretch.

4 / Repeat on the other side.

SCAPULA/DELT STRETCH (C)

1 / Assume a standing position and draw your right arm across your body.

2 / Grip your elbow with your hand in front of your upper abs (selecting an overhand grip this time).

3 / Apply pressure across/towards your body with your left hand until you feel a stretch through your back/shoulders/traps.

4 / Keep your palm facing behind you and thumb upwards throughout.

5 / Repeat on the other side.

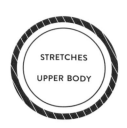

HANGING BACK STRETCH

1 / Place both hands on the arm of a sofa or back of a stable chair.

2 / With your feet shoulder width apart allow your knees to bend slightly, enough to allow for a small arch in your back.

3 / Push your chest towards the floor (and sit back) until you feel a stretch through the lats.

4 / You may also complete this with one arm by gripping a doorframe and applying pressure backwards in addition to the gravitational downwards hang.

5 / Repeat on the other side.

STANDING TRAPS STRETCH (A)

1 / Assume a standing position with your arms by your side.

2 / Push your right palm towards the floor and tilt your head to the left.

3 / Do this until you feel a stretch through your neck/traps.

4 / Repeat on the other side.

STANDING TRAPS STRETCH (B)

1 / Assume a standing position with your arms by your side.

2 / Aim to touch your chin to your sternum and allow your upper spine to flex and shoulders to round slightly, doing so until you feel a stretch through the entire trapezius (from the base of your head to around halfway down your spinal column).

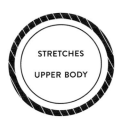

SEATED TRAPS STRETCH

1 / Sit in a wooden dining chair with your pelvis tilted forwards enough to allow for good posture to be assumed.

2 / With your chest proud and shoulders held back slightly, grip under the edge of the chair seat with your right hand, while keeping your arm straight (elbow extended).

3 / Lean away from your right hand and tilt your head to the left until you feel a stretch through your neck/traps.

4 / Repeat on the other side.

TRICEP (AND LAT) STRETCH

1 / Assume a standing position and extend your right arm directly upright.

2 / Flex your elbow and try to touch your fingertips to your left rear deltoid muscle.

3 / Grip your right elbow with your left hand and apply pressure by gently pulling your elbow across the rear of your body.

4 / Do this until you feel a stretch through your tricep and back muscles. You may lean your torso to the left to increase the stretch.

5 / Repeat on the other side.

BICEP STRETCH

1 / Stand at a right angle to a wall or a closed door.

2 / Extend your right arm horizontally outwards from your shoulder and place your palm on the wall with your fingertips pointing downwards.

3 / Attempt to get the hand flat against the wall while keeping your arm fully extended, but if you feel a stretch strongly before this do not force it as you may cause damage to your elbow/bicep and wrist joint.

4 / Repeat on the other side.

FOREARM STRETCH

1 / Assume a standing position and extend both arms out in front of you.

2 / With your right palm facing away from your body, and fingertips pointing upwards, grip the fingers/top of your hand and apply pressure back towards your body.

3 / Try to keep your elbow straight and apply enough pressure to feel a stretch through the forearm.

4 / Repeat on the other side.

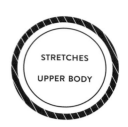
SHOULDER STRETCH

1 / Assume a standing position by an open doorway.

2 / Place your right arm on the doorframe.

3 / Keep your upper arm horizontal to the ground and forearm (elbow to fingertips) flat on the doorframe.

4 / Step through the door, ensuring your chest stays pointing forwards, as if you were walking straight through the door (don't let your left shoulder start to round the door and point towards the right).

5 / You should feel a stretch through your upper chest and shoulders, and may turn away from the right shoulder to increase this.

6 / Repeat on the other side.

CHEST STRETCH

1 / Assume a standing position beside an open door.

2 / Place the base of your right hand on the doorframe and step through the door, keeping your arm fully extended.

3 / Turn your torso to the left to increase the stretch (and ensure your left shoulder does not turn towards the right).

4 / Repeat on both sides.

PARTNER-ASSISTED CHEST STRETCH

1 / Assume a standing position and place your hands on your lower back, with your fingertips touching your lower spine, and thumbs hooked over/on top of your hips.

2 / Allow your partner to place their hands on the outside of your elbows and apply pressure inwards across your spine.

3 / Let them know when you want them to stop applying more pressure, and get them to hold the enforced stretch for 20–30 seconds.

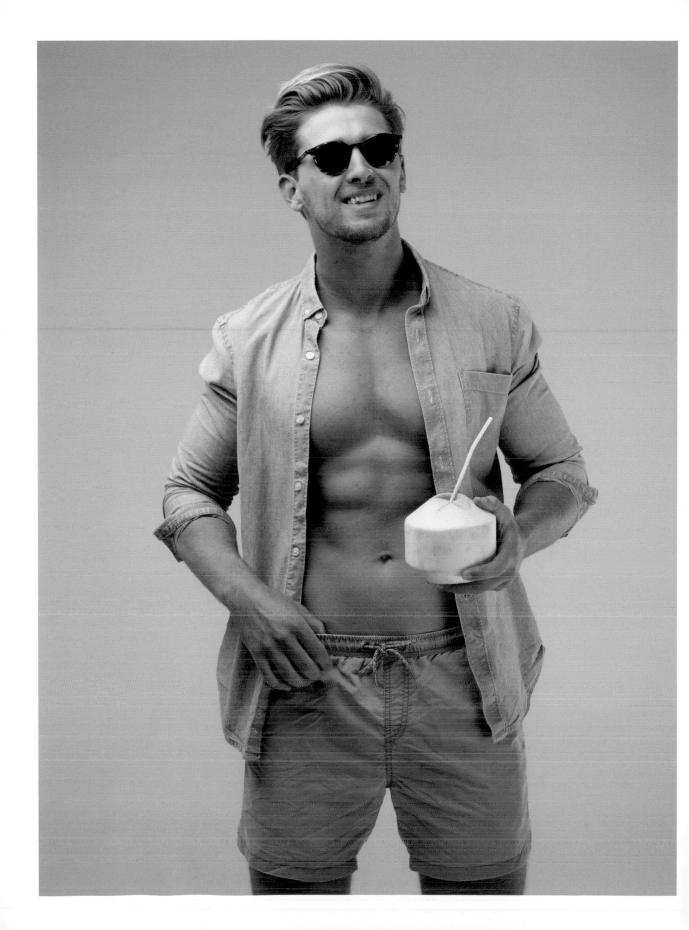

STRONGER

||||||||||||||||||||||||||||||||||||||||||||||||||||||||||||||||||||

Training your body also means training your mind. We at LDNM take a holistic approach to working out – it's not just about what you eat and how you train, it's also about getting your mind in the right space so that negative feelings and thoughts don't distract you from your decision to get Leaner, Fitter, Stronger.

The good news is that you've made a positive choice in wanting to change. Change is such an optimistic idea – you want to change your body to ensure that it does the things that you want it to do for as long as possible. You want to feel better in your clothes, or become more flexible. Whatever your reasons for change, you need to try to harness that initial optimism so that it carries you towards your weight-loss or muscle-building journey, whatever road blocks you meet along the way.

This chapter will help you do just that.

There's a reason Lloyd is wearing sunglasses and holding a coconut. We want you to embrace the fun side, the happy side and the living-life-to-the-full side of getting fit and healthy. Now channel your inner Lloyd: go grab your coconut.

WILLPOWER VS PERSEVERANCE
||||||||||||||||||||||||||||||||||||||||||||||||||

A lot of people come to us and say that they've tried other diets and fitness programmes and that they haven't had the willpower to see them through. Why should they try something new when clearly they haven't managed to finish what they started? In other words: why should our programme help them when they've failed so many times before?

This is what the idea of willpower does. If you haven't been able to achieve the results you want, you've not just failed, you've shown yourself to be 'lacking in character'. So that's one more thing to beat yourself up about.

Let's knock that on the head right away. Willpower is a short-term solution to a short-term problem. It's not sustainable in the long run. Perseverance, on the other hand, is kinder. It says 'If I haven't done well today, if I keep trying I may do better tomorrow'. Perseverance is made up of the small increments of positive actions you do every day that result in achieving your end goal. Everyone who's completed a difficult challenge or a long-term goal did so because of perseverance, not willpower.

Take learning to drive, for instance. Your end goal is getting your driver's licence. But remember all the stages that you had to go through in order to achieve that goal. You had to study for and pass the theory test. You had to learn to check the mirrors, parallel-park and take the right approach to roundabouts. Then, when you were ready, came the test itself. You may not have passed the first time, but perseverance made you try again. It wasn't willpower that got you your driver's licence; it was perseverance.

Let's have a look at why you might 'fail' when it comes to weight loss, and why that has little to do with willpower.

First of all, diets that restrict you from eating a certain food group, whether it's carbs or fat, are doomed to fail. As we've said on page 39 [diet section], this is because all food groups have their place on your plate.

Secondly, restrictive diets aren't very much fun. You might find yourself declining invitations because you're worried you might eat or drink more than you wanted. Or you might go out with your friends and feel miserable that you're not able to eat and drink what they're having. Or you go out and overeat and drink much more than usual and feel terrible the next day.

Thirdly, as we've said before, human beings are often drawn to what they can't have. It's the 'pink elephant' theory. Try not to think of a pink elephant. Right? We bet you have a pink elephant image in your head right now. You've decided to cut cake completely out of your diet? We bet you think a lot more about cake than you would if you allowed yourself a piece of cake now and again. And what happens when you decide you can't have something is that – more often than not – you end up bingeing on it, which makes you doubt your willpower.

Thinking of yourself as having willpower is, in the long run, not very useful. Instead, what you need to do is create conditions that make it easy for you to follow the programme. This means setting one clear goal, breaking it up into smaller, more achievable, goals and rewarding yourself when you meet them, like you did when you were learning to drive a car. We want you to think in terms of perseverance, not in terms of having willpower or not. If you persevere with something, you keep on with it, even if you've had a day or two when you've not followed the programme. That's fine – don't beat yourself up about it – just make sure to keep your final goal in your sights.

MARGINAL GAINS

|||||||||||||||||||||||||||||||||||||||||||||||||

The year of the London Olympics, 2012, was when the idea of marginal gains became part of the public's consciousness. Bradley Wiggins, riding for Sky and Team GB, had a phenomenal year, winning Paris–Nice, the Tour de Romandie, the Critérium du Dauphiné, and the world's most prestigious and well-known cycling event, the Tour de France, becoming the first Briton to do so. He also won gold at the Olympics, Time Trial and was recognised for his remarkable achievements by being awarded the British Sportsperson of the Year.

Wiggins achieved that success due to the principle of 'marginal gains', which was put in place in Team GB and Sky by sports director Dave Brailsford. Marginal gains means small improvements you make across a wide range of areas. Famously, Brailsford retaught his team to wash their hands more thoroughly in order to improve their chances of not getting sick. Marginal gains took British cycling to the very pinnacle of the sport.

You don't need to be as committed to the principle of marginal gains as the members of British cycling, but you can use the idea to help make small improvements to your lifestyle that will help you become Leaner, Fitter and Stronger. These could include:

- Instead of watching that TV show you're not that bothered by, spend that time preparing packed lunches for the week.
- Set your alarm half an hour earlier and have a good breakfast that sets you up for the day.
- Get off the bus or the Tube a couple of stops from your destination and walk the rest of the way.
- Carry a bottle of water with you at all times to remain hydrated. It's also useful to have a drink handy as often the body mistakes thirst for hunger.
- Keep healthy snacks in your desk drawer at work to eat when you're feeling peckish.
- Invest in the best pair of training shoes you can afford. Women: wear the most supportive sports bra you can find.
- Spend ten minutes in the evening reflecting on your day.

" Stop saying
'I cant' and
start saying
'I will' "

KEEPING UP MOTIVATION

||||||||||||||||||||||||||||||||||||||||||||||||

When you start a fitness programme, you're raring to go. You start off positively – 'I've got this' – and it's easy to make healthy choices when it comes to food because you've got that burst of energy that comes with starting something new. You're highly motivated, and that's great – you should use that initial drive to push you through the first stages of your fitness programme.

But what to do when you're a few weeks or months down the track? Do you find your concentration starting to wander? Are you sticking to your programme as closely as you were in the beginning, or are you making excuses not to do your exercises or go to the gym?

You're not going to achieve the results you want overnight. It's going to take weeks or months. You need to find strategies to keep your motivation high. We know how difficult it is to push through an hour at the gym when we're not feeling it, but we also know how exercise feels when we're looking forward to it.

So how do you keep up the motivation?

INTRINSIC VS EXTRINSIC MOTIVATION

|||||||||||||||||||||||||||||||||||||||||||||||||

Look back on some of your achievements – they don't need to be fitness-based, they can be anything where you've needed to put in a sustained amount of effort over a significant period of time. You could look at the motivation it took for you to complete your degree, or finish a personal project. Can you identify what drove you the most? Was it the piece of paper you received at the end with your name on it? Was it graduating in front of your friends and family? Was it the sense of achievement you felt? Perhaps it was all three. But try to identify what it was that motivated you the most.

INTRINSIC MOTIVATION

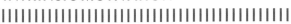

Intrinsic motivation means that you are motivated to achieve because of how it makes you feel inside, or internally. You are motivated because you like the feeling you get when you reach a goal. You don't need an external award or congratulations (although it's a nice added bonus) because you know you've done well.

ADVANTAGES OF INTRINSIC MOTIVATION

- You're self-starting.
- You don't need rewards to get motivated – you can rely on yourself.
- Process is important, rather than results, making you more likely to stick with you.

DISADVANTAGES OF INTRINSIC MOTIVATION

- You risk becoming complacent and don't push yourself hard enough.
- Success can be harder to measure whether you're relying on how it makes you feel.

HOW TO KEEP MOTIVATION HIGH WHEN YOU'RE INTRINSICALLY MOTIVATED

If you're intrinsically motivated, once you decide to work out or change your eating plan, you should be able to keep to it because you find motivation within yourself, you don't need any external rewards to keep you on track.

However, make sure that you keep pushing yourself and don't become complacent. You could introduce a competitive element to your training by working out with a friend.

EXTRINSIC MOTIVATION

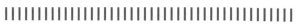

Extrinsic motivation means that you are motivated to achieve because of some external rewards, such as money, prizes or praise. It's likely that most of us are more extrinsically motivated than we are intrinsically.

ADVANTAGES OF EXTRINSIC MOTIVATION

- You have a concrete measure of achievement.
- Working towards a reward gives you an added incentive to achieve.
- When motivation is low, you're more able to stick to the programme as you know you'll get a reward at the end of it.

DISADVANTAGES OF EXTRINSIC MOTIVATION

- If you don't receive the reward or acknowledgement of your achievement, it can make you feel bad.
- Results become more important than process, which means you can lose motivation if don't get the results you want when you want them.

HOW TO KEEP MOTIVATION HIGH WHEN YOU'RE EXTRINSICALLY MOTIVATED

Introducing rewards into your training regimen is a great idea to keep your motivation high. Make both the rewards and the goal specific. Break up your large goal into smaller ones and reward yourself each time you hit a goal. Perhaps pop 50p into a piggy bank each time you work out – when it's full you can treat yourself to something you really want. You could indulge in a spa treatment once you've lost a certain amount of weight, or a set of new training clothes.

CHECKING IN WITH YOUR GOALS

||||||||||||||||||||||||||||||||||||||||||||||||||

Every now and then it's a good idea to check in with your goals to see how you're doing and where you are on your journey to a healthier you. Take some time to do this – an hour or so – when you're alone and likely to be undisturbed. Now would be a good time to look at your progress selfies. You're not just losing fat or gaining muscle, you're changing your body shape, and having those progress selfies are going to help you see how far you've come.

Take some time to think about your goals. If you want to lose fat, for instance, how much more do you need to lose? Perhaps you had a set weight goal in mind, but with your new diet and exercise plan, you realise that your body is looking the way you want it to, and you decide now's the time to maintain your current weight. Or, perhaps, you're not gaining muscle as fast as you'd like, so now's a good time to go over your plan, check your TDEE and your surplus calories. With your increased activity level, are you eating enough? Whatever stage you are at, taking some time out to check in with your goals will help you achieve the body you want.

We love to see progress shots, so when you're ready, please share them on Twitter (@LDN_Muscle) or on Instagram (@ldn_muscle) using the hashtag #Leanfitstrong.

UPDATE YOUR PLAYLIST

This might seem like a trivial thing to do, but it's not. For a lot of us, music provides the rhythm to our training. If you're bored with your music choice, chances are you may get bored with your training regime. Changing up your playlist to new tunes or old classics will help keep your motivation high.

And don't forget – you can have as many different playlists as you like – perhaps you have one for legs and abs and another for when you're doing cardio. It's up to you!

PLATEAUS

||||||||||||||||||||||||||||||||||||||||||||||

You started off great. You worked hard and stuck to your fitness and eating programme. You started to see results, you're motivated and everything is going well.

But now you're a few weeks or months in. You're still working hard, but you're stuck. You just don't seem to be shifting the weight or building the muscles as you used to.

You've hit a plateau. A plateau is when you're putting in the work, but the results seem to have stalled. Most people hit a plateau during their fitness journey, but that doesn't mean that they don't suck. The good news is that plateaus are just a stage that you can move past. They offer you an opportunity to take a look at your programme and see if it's still working for you.

HOW TO MOVE PAST A PLATEAU

||||||||||||||||||||||||||||||||||||||||||||||

- Check your food planner and be honest with yourself – are you sticking to it as much as you were at the beginning of your programme? Is lethargy kicking in because of your food choices?
- Check your training programme – is it time to move up to the next level?
- Go for a wider range of exercises – this will hit your muscles and body in a different way it isn't used to, and the change in movement should spur you on mentally too.
- Remember to rest, listen to your body and understand the difference between DOMS and injury! Take rest weeks off completely from weights training every couple of months if you feel you need a mental and physical break, and ensure you don't skip rest days.
- Train with a different partner – this is not to say that you have to turn your back on your loyal exercise buddy, but mixing it up is a great way to get past a plateau.
- Are you getting enough sleep? Insufficient sleep can limit fat loss.
- Check your stress levels. External stress can hamper training and your body's ability to lose fat and gain muscle, so remember to make time to relax and decompress.

FITTING FITNESS INTO WORK AND SOCIAL LIFE

||||||||||||||||||||||||||||||||||||||||||||||||||

Diets that are too restrictive, or workout schedules that are too strenuous or stringent are unsustainable in the long term as they are difficult to maintain if you want to go out with your friends now and again, or even fit in training around your job. It can start to feel like you're punishing yourself for not being in the shape you want, and that's demoralising.

We want you to enjoy your new training programme and enjoy your food. We want you to go out for a meal with your friends without stressing about carbohydrates. In fact, it's absolutely essential that you maintain your social life. We're advocating a lifestyle change, not a short-term restrictive diet or overambitious training regime. Having fun with family and friends is important – and sometimes that involves meals out, and yes, alcohol. Here are some tips:

GOING OUT

||||||||||||||||||||||||||||||||||||||||||||||||||

- Some types of cuisines fit into a healthy diet more easily than others. Mexican food, for example, can be very healthy if you cut down on the cheese. Choose foods cooked in the tandoori oven if you're going out for an Indian curry. Italian food is great if you choose tomato-based sauces rather than creamy ones.

- If you're running a calorie deficit, eat fewer calories during the day, but don't let yourself get hungry. If you're too hungry before a meal, you're more likely to binge and go over your calorie target.

- Low-to-moderate intake of alcohol has been shown to have health benefits. We think alcohol is fine, in moderation, and obviously don't drink every night or before a workout. Take account of the calories in each drink you have and factor them into your daily calorie allowance.

- If you do go overboard on food or alcohol, don't beat yourself up about it. Start the next day afresh. As long as you don't make a habit of it, the odd big night out isn't going to affect your training programme too badly.

We know how difficult it is to fit in training around work demands and long commutes. Here are a few tips:

- Get up early and train in the morning. Early morning is a great time to go to the gym as it avoids the peak at the end of your day and means that it's likely you'll get all the equipment to yourself. It also sets you up for the day, and you're more likely to follow your food plan and training programmes if you start your day off well. Make sure to eat afterwards – take a protein shake with you to drink on your commute to work if you haven't got time to prep food. We aren't saying that getting out of bed early is easy, particularly when it's dark outside, but just remind yourself – it will be worth it!

- There are a couple of downsides to working out in the early morning: at the start you may be battling with tiredness, and your social life might suffer a little if you've been up since 5am, and your buddies want to party into the night. Make sure that you have something healthy to eat around 2 or 3pm so that you don't hit that wall of tiredness.

- If you can't work out in the early morning, try getting out of the office at lunchtime. If you have a park near by, try some of the gym-free training suggestions in the Fitter section (see pages 153–257).

- If you've worked late, you can still fit in some training using our suggestions in the Fitter section – try one of the gymfree circuits that be done at home.

REMEMBER

The key to a healthy lifestyle and sustainable progress in your health and fitness goals is finding balance in your work, social and home life.

VISUALISATION

||||||||||||||||||||||||||||||||||||||||||||

Visualisation is a technique used by sportspeople to imagine a challenge and then overcome it. Jessica Ennis-Hill uses visualisation to create the image of the perfect technique in her head; on the night before a match Andy Murray goes to the court he'll be playing at and visualises his success. Visualisation is a powerful tool that can go hand in hand with training. Using your imagination to show you how it looks and feels to have achieved your ideal physique can really help you achieve it.

HOW TO USE VISUALISATION

|||||||||||||||||||||||||||||||||||||||||||||

Choose a time and a place where you can relax for a few minutes without any distractions. Turn off notifications on your phone. Lie back, or sit, in a comfortable position. Think about your goal. Once it's clear in your mind, relax, close your eyes and let yourself visualise yourself having achieved your goal.

Where are you?
What do you look like?
What are you wearing?
How do you feel?
Who are you with?

Try and be as specific as possible. Engage all your senses. Perhaps you're on a beach with the wind in your hair, the sun beating down upon your shoulders and you can smell the sea. Think of what you're wearing. Think of yourself as your ideal size, running towards the water. Or you might think of yourself mountain biking a course in Scotland or going out with friends to a new club. Whatever scenario you choose, really try to inhabit it and experience it through all your senses.

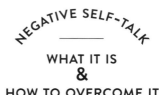

NEGATIVE SELF-TALK

WHAT IT IS
&
HOW TO OVERCOME IT

Constructive criticism is a good thing; it takes account of your
strengths and weaknesses and offers advice to make you better.
However, not many of us criticise ourselves constructively. Instead
we are too harsh on ourselves, overlooking our strengths in favour
of focusing on our weaknesses and blowing them up out of
all proportion.

Negative self-talk is damaging to your mood and to your
motivation. If you are always focusing on your weaknesses and your
failures rather than your strengths and successes, then you are
setting yourself up to fail in the long term. Remember, we all fail
from time to time, it's not just part of life, it's also a great tool for
learning. But it's just as important to focus on your successes.

If you find yourself engaging in negative self-talk,
here's a few things that you can do to try and squash down
that super-critical voice.

Go outside and do some exercise.
We don't mean a full-on HIIT or weight-training session, unless
that's part of your weekly plan, but a brisk walk outside can work
wonders.

Imagine what your negative self-talk voice looks like,
and make it say its criticisms in a funny-sounding voice.
Picture slamming the door on it, or forcing it inside a strongbox,
locking it and throwing away the key.

Argue with your self-talk.
If it says something like 'why bother going to the gym? They're
all hard bodies there; you're going to look out of place' tell it
'everyone started somewhere, and I'm going to focus on myself,
my sets and repetitions'.

Ask yourself whether you would say what you say
to yourself to your best friend?
You wouldn't, would you? So why say it to yourself?
Love your imperfections. We all have them. And sometimes
they're the things our family and friends love about us the most.

But most of all, be kind to yourself, show as much empathy
to yourself as you do to others, and don't let the negative
self-talk win.

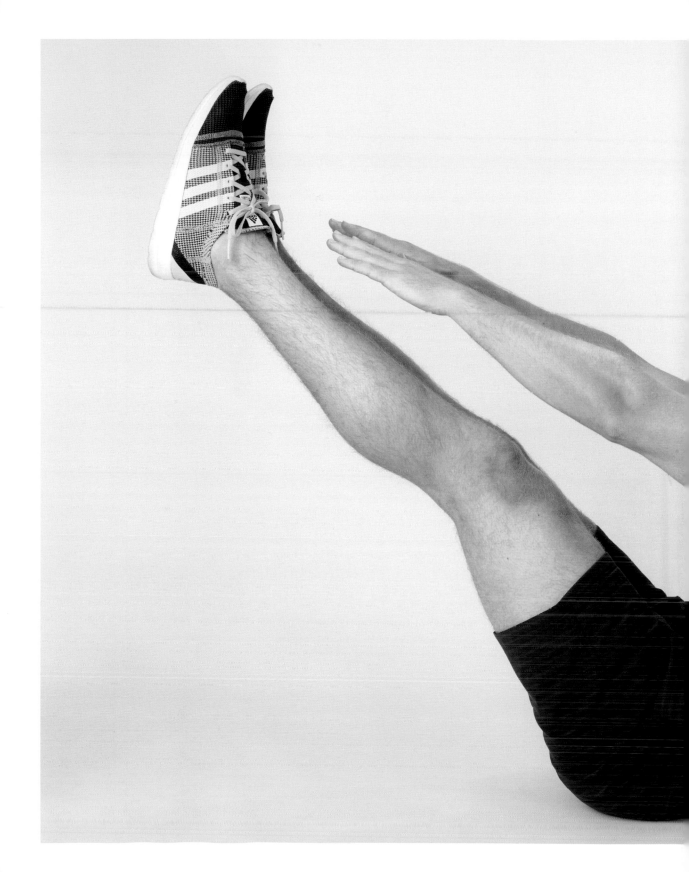

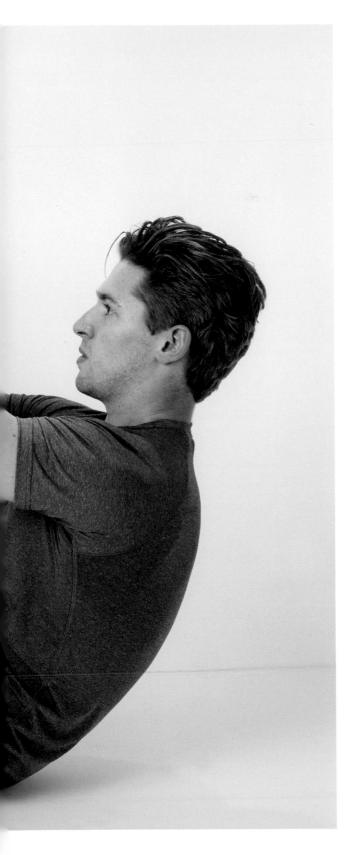

TRACKING YOUR PROGRESS

There are many ways to track your progress – from apps that you can use on your phone, like My Fitness Pal, to going analogue – with a planner like the one overleaf. It doesn't matter which kind of trainer you go for, the main thing is that you are keeping your fitness goal in sight (and in mind). Here are some templates to get you started.

	MONDAY	**TUESDAY**	**WEDNESDAY**
	date	date	date

GOAL _____ _____ _____

TDEE _____ _____ _____

FOOD

Breakfast

Snack

Lunch

Snack

Dinner

Water

TRAINING *Today I* _____ *Today I* _____ *Today I* _____

MOOD
circle your mood   ☠ ★ ★★ ★★★   ☠ ★ ★★ ★★★   ☠ ★ ★★ ★★★

GOAL

THURSDAY

date

FRIDAY

date

SATURDAY

date

SUNDAY

date

Today I

Today I

Today I

Today I

☠ ★ ★★ ★★★ ☠ ★ ★★ ★★★ ☠ ★ ★★ ★★★ ☠ ★ ★★ ★★★

	MONDAY	TUESDAY	WEDNESDAY
	date	date	date
GOAL			
TDEE			
FOOD			
Breakfast			
Snack			
Lunch			
Snack			
Dinner			
Water			
TRAINING	Today I	Today I	Today I
MOOD *circle your mood*	☠ ★ ★★ ★★★	☠ ★ ★★ ★★★	☠ ★ ★★ ★★★
GOAL			

THURSDAY

date

FRIDAY

date

SATURDAY

date

SUNDAY

date

Today I

☠ ★ ★★ ★★★

Today I

☠ ★ ★★ ★★★

Today I

☠ ★ ★★ ★★★

Today I

☠ ★ ★★ ★★★

GOAL TRACKER

___ date

S — SPECIFIC

M — MEASURABLE

A — ACTION-ORIENTATED

R — REALISTIC

T — TIME-BASED

Index

Page references in *italics*
indicate photographs.

A

abdominal stretch 247
  prone abdominal stretch 248
abs workouts 203–6, 226–31,
  240–1
  *see also under individual
  exercise*
activity factor, find your 24–5
advanced workout day 234–43
  1: legs & back 234–5
  2: chests & shoulders 236–7
  3: back & arms 238 9
  4: leg & abs 240–1
  5: full body 242–3
angry cat 248
any-fish traybake 112, *113*
apple & blackberry crumble
  139, *140, 141*
arnold press 222
avo-choc truffles 138

B

back workouts:
  back & arms workout 238–9
  chest, back & arms workout
    232–3
  hamstrings, back, biceps
    workout 218–21
  legs & back workout 234–5
  *see also under individual
  exercise*
'bad' foods 33, 35, 40, 153
baked tomato with kale &
  goat's cheese 48, *49*
bananas:
  banana & chocolate (n)ice
    cream 126, *127*
  banana bread 128
barbell:
  barbell curls 233
  barbell curls superset to
    skull crushers 239

barbell squats 227, 240
  reverse barbell curls 221
  stiff-leg barbell deadlifts
    226, *226*
BCAAs (branched chain amino
  acids) 38
beef:
  beef ramen 90, *91*
  beef tagine 101
beetroot, goat's cheese & rocket
  tart 151
beginner workout 203–17
  day 1: lower body (legs & abs)
    203–6
  day 2: upper body 207–13
  day 3: full-body circuits
    214–17
bench:
  bench dips 184, *184*
  bench press 222, 236
  bench press-ups 185, *185*
  decline bench press 232
bent over row 171, 172, *172,
  173, 173*, 232
berry bomb smoothie 50, *51*
bicep curls 211, *211*, 214, 215,
  215
bicep stretch 252
bicycle crunches 178, 179, *179,*
  188
BMR (Basal Metabolic Rate)
  23–4
body fat 20, 23, 24, 25, 26
body weight squats 189, *189*
breakfast 44–60
brownies:
  fudge protein 146
  sweet potato 129
buddy training 195–201
  medicine ball slam passes
    200, *200*
  plank challenge 197, *197*
  press-up challenge 196, *196*
  Russian twist and pass 199,
    199

shuttle runs, tag & go 201,
  201
sit-ups passing medicine ball
  198, *198*
stair runs, tag & go 201, *201*
Bulgarian split squats 228, 229
bulking, training and 29
burgers:
  burger with wings & lemon
    'mayo' 104, 105
  inside-out burger, the 102,
    103
  vegan burger, the best 86, *87*
burpees 174, *174*, 243
butternut squash, stuffed 98, *99*

C

caffeine 37
calf:
  calf extension 241
  calf stretch 246
caramelised red onion soup 63
carbohydrates 14, 28, 35, 37, 39,
  41, 155, 262
cardio myths 155
carrot & walnut muffins 124
cauliflower:
  cheesy cauliflower fritters
    76, *77*
  pumpkin & cauliflower curry
    85
cheat day 41, 42
cheat meal 28
cheesy cauliflower fritters 76,
  77
chest stretch 253
chest workouts:
  chest & shoulders workout
    236–7
  chest, back & arms workout
    232–3
  chest, triceps & shoulders
    workout 222–5
  *see also under individual
  exercise*

chicken:
chicken enchiladas 93
chicken korma soup 71
coronation chicken 78
curried chicken scotch eggs
52
easy-peasy chicken pie 144,
145
soy sesame chicken &
cucumber salad 66, *67*
chilli no-carne 84
chocolate:
banana & chocolate (n)ice
cream 126, *127*
chocolate coconut cookies
142
chocolate orange pots 134,
135
ultimate chocolate proats 54
'clean diet' 41
clean eating 28
cod with aubergine fries, crispy
106, *107*
commando 169, *169*
commandos superset to
alternating lunges 187
cooking every meal 40
cookies, chocolate coconut 142
Coronation chicken 78
courgette & feta frittata
muffins 120, *121*
cream cheese, smoked salmon
& spinach tart 149
creatine (creapure) 37
crispy cod with aubergine fries
106, *107*
cross-trainer 158
crumble, apple & blackberry
139, *140, 141*
crunches:
crunches superset to Russian
twists 204, *205*
feet raised weighted
crunches 230
knee in crunches 191, *191*

sofa crunches 194, *194*
step ups superset to bicycle
crunches 188
curried chicken scotch eggs 52
curried sweet potato & ginger
soup 64
curry, pumpkin & cauliflower
85
cutting, training 29

D

DB shrugs 235, 238
deadlifts 234, 242
kettlebell deadlift 175, *175*
stiff-leg barbell deadlifts
226, *226*
stiff-leg deadlifts 218, 240
decline bench press 232
dietary keywords, acronyms
and buzzwords decoded 28
dinners 80–115
DOMS ('delayed onset muscle
soreness') 29, 261
drop set 182
dumbbell:
dumbbell chest press 210,
210, 242
dumbbell hammer curls 220,
220
dumbbell hammer shoulder
press 208, *208*
dumbbell lateral raises 209,
209, 223
incline dumbbell press 222,
233, 236
single-arm dumbbell row 219
squat and dumbbell press 177,
177
standing dumbbell shoulder
press 236

E

easy-peasy chicken pie 144, 145
easy-peasy sushi 70
80–20 rule 41

eggs Benedict omelette 53
enchiladas, chicken 93
energy booster smoothie 50, *51*
erector spine stretch 247
extrinsic motivation 258, 259
EZ bar skull crushers 224, *224*

F

failure, training 29
fat loss 23, 25, 38, 155
feet raised weighted crunches
230
fitter 152–253
buddy training 195–201
gym training 202–43
gym-free workouts 182–94
HIIT 29, 155, 156–61
myth busting 154–5
stretches 244–53
tabata circuits 162–81
TDEE 154
flexible dieting 28, 39
food grinder roast with sweet
potato dauphinoise, The 108,
109, 110
forearm stretch 252
form/technique, training 29
4-ingredient heroes 143–7
freezer 43
French toast, PB&J 58, 59
fridge 43
frittata:
courgette & feta frittata
muffins 120, *121*
sweet potato frittata 147
fritters, cheesy cauliflower 76,
77
fudge protein brownies 146

G

gains, training 29
gingerbread protein shake
smoothie 50, *51*
glute bridges 190, *190*
glute stretch 245

goals:
    checking in with your 260
    set your 27
    smart goals 27
    your goal 28
goblet squats 204, *205*
going out 262–3
'good' vs 'bad' foods 35
granola pots, homemade 55
Green One smoothie, The 50, *51*
groin stretch 246
gym training 202–43
    advanced workout day 1: legs
        & back 234–5
        exercise 1: deadlifts 234
        exercise 2: lat pull down
            234
        exercise 3: leg press 234
        exercise 4: seated cable row
            235
        exercise 5: hamstring curls
            235
        exercise 6: DB shrugs 235
    advanced workout day 2:
        chests & shoulders 236–7
        exercise 1: bench press 236
        exercise 2: standing
            dumbbell shoulder press
            236
        exercise 3: incline
            dumbbell press 236
        exercise 4: upright rows
            237
        exercise 5: plate squeeze
            raises superset to front
            plate raise 237
    advanced workout day 3:
        back & arms 238–9
        exercise 1: lat pulldown
            238
        exercise 2: seated cable
            rows 238
        exercise 3: straight arm
            pull downs 238
        exercise 4: DB shrugs 238

exercise 5: barbell curls
    superset to skull crushers
    239
exercise 6: tricep kickbacks
    239
advanced workout day 4: leg
    & abs 240–1
    exercise 1: barbell squats
        240
    exercise 2: leg press 240
    exercise 3: stiff-leg
        deadlifts 240
    exercise 4: hamstring curls
        241
    exercise 5: quad extension
        241
    exercise 6: calf extension
        241
advanced workout day 5: full
    body 242–3
    exercise 1: deadlifts 242
    exercise 2: dumbbell chest
        press 242
    exercise 3: lat pulldown
        242
    exercise 4: military press
        242
    exercise 5: skull crushers
        superset to hammer curls
        243
    exercise 6: burpees 243
beginner workout day 1:
    lower body (legs & abs)
    203–6
    exercise 1: quad extension
        203
    exercise 2: hamstring curls
        203
    exercise 3: leg press 203
    exercise 4: goblet squats
        204, *205*
    exercise 5: crunches
        superset to Russian
        twists 204, *205*
    exercise 6: planks 206, *206*

beginner workout day 2:
    upper body 207–13
    exercise 1: lat pulldown
        207
    exercise 2: seated cable row
        207
    exercise 3: dumbbell
        hammer shoulder press
        208, *208*
    exercise 4: dumbbell lateral
        raises 209, *209*
    exercise 5: dumbbell chest
        press 210, *210*
    exercise 6: bicep curls 211,
        211
    exercise 7: press ups 212,
        212, 213
beginner workout day 3: full
    body circuits 214–17
    circuit 1 214–15
        bicep curls 215, *215*
        lateral raises 215, *215*
        plank 214, *214*
        squat press 214, *214*
    circuit 2 216–17
        kettlebell swings 217, *217*
        press ups 217, *217*
        squat thrusts 216, *216*
        triceps extensions 216,
            216
intermediate workout day 1:
    hamstrings, back, biceps
    218–21
    exercise 1: stiff leg
        deadlifts 218
    exercise 2: hamstring curls
        218
    exercise 3: lat pull-down
        218
    exercise 4: single arm
        dumbbell row 219
    exercise 5: straight arm
        pull down 219
    exercise 6: dumbbell
        hammer curls 220

exercise 7: zottman curls 221

exercise 8: reverse barbell curls 221

intermediate workout day 2: chest, triceps & shoulders 222–5

exercise 1: bench press 222

exercise 2: arnold press 222

exercise 3: incline dumbbell press 222

exercise 4: dumbbell lateral raises 223

exercise 5: EZ bar skull crushers 224, *224*

exercise 6: tricep pull downs 225

exercise 7: tricep kickbacks 225

intermediate workout day 3: legs & abs 226–31

exercise 1: stiff leg barbell deadlifts 226, *226*

exercise 2: quad extension 227

exercise 3: barbell squats 227

exercise 4: hamstring curls 228

exercise 5: Bulgarian split squats 228, 229

exercise 6: feet raised weighted crunches 230

exercise 7: laying leg raises 230, 231

exercise 8: Russian twists 230

intermediate workout day 4: chest, back & arms 232–3

exercise 1: bent over row 232

exercise 2: decline bench press 232

exercise 3: lat pull down 232

exercise 4: incline dumbbell press 233

exercise 5: barbell curls 233

exercise 6: tricep rope pull downs 233

gym-free workouts 182–94

drop set 182

6-12-25 182

superset 182

workout 1: park bench 183, *183*

exercise 1: single-leg step up 183, *183*

exercise 2: bench dips 184, *184*

exercise 3: bench press-ups 185, *185*

exercise 4: mountain climbers (hands raised) 186, *186*

workout 2: outdoors 187

body weight squats 189, *189*

circuit 3: static lunges/ squats/glute 189

exercise 1: squat jumps superset to press ups 187

exercise 2: commandos superset to alternating lunges 187

exercise 3: step ups superset to bicycle crunches 188

glute bridges 190, *190*

static lunge 189, *189*

workout 3: sofa workout 191–4, *191*

exercise 1: knee in crunches 191, *191*

exercise 2: sofa dips 192, *192*

exercise 3: mountain climbers (hands raised) 193, *193*

exercise 4: sofa crunches 194, *194*

H

hamstring curls 203, 218, 228, 235, 241

hamstring stretch 245

hanging back stretch 251

high knees 163, *163*

HIIT 20, 27, 29, 155, 156–61, 265

workout 1: static bike pyramid 157

workout 2: cross-trainer 158

workout 3: treadmill 159

workout 4: rowing 160

workout 5: swimming 161

workouts 157

hip flexor stretch 246

hip/oblique stretch 247

homemade granola pots 55

honey fruit and oat bars 60

huevos rancheros 46, *47*

hummus 4 ways 118, *119*

I

ice cream 39

banana & chocolate (n)ice cream 126, *127*

pistachio 132, *133*

IIFYM (eating anything you want, so long as it hits your macros) 28

incline dumbbell press 222, 233, 236

inside-out burger, the 102, *103*

instant oats 37

intermediate workout 218–33

day 1: hamstrings, back, biceps 218–21

day 2: chest, triceps & shoulders 222–5

day 3: legs & abs 226–31

day 4: chest, back & arms 232–3

intrinsic motivation 258, 259

intrinsic vs extrinsic motivation 258

J

James 17, *18*

K

kettlebell:
deadlift 174, 175, *175*
swings 216, 217, *217*
keywords, acronyms and buzzwords 28–9
knee-in crunches 191, *191*
kneeling back stretch 249

L

lamb meatballs, spicy 94, *95*
lat pulldown 207, 218, 232, 234, 238, 242
lateral raises 214, 215, *215*
dumbbell lateral raises 209, *209*, 223
laying leg raises 167, 170, *170*, 230, 231
LDNM 10, 11
leaner 33–43
flexible dieting 28, 39
'good' vs 'bad' foods 35
myth busting 39–42, 154–5
stocking up 43
supplements 36–8, 155
track your week 34
leek, blue cheese & bacon tart 148
leg press 203, 234, 240
legs workouts:
legs & abs workout 203–6, 226–31, 240–1
legs & back workout 234–5
see also under individual exercise
lemon polenta cake 130, *131*
Lloyd *12*, 13
lower body:
(legs & abs) workout 203–6

stretches 245–7
lunch 61–79

M

macros 17, 20, 26, 28, 36
marginal gains 257
marinated tofu stir-fry 88, *89*
Max 14, *15*, 7, 72, 76
measuring your progress 22
meatballs, spicy lamb 94, *95*
medicine ball slam passes 200, *200*
Mexican layer bowl 68, 69
military press 178, 180, *180*, 242
Moroccan pizza 82, *83*
motivation 258, 259
mountain climber 167, 168, *168*
(Hands Raised) 186, *186*, 193, *193*
muffins:
carrot & walnut 124
courgette & feta frittata muffins 120, *121*
multivitamin 38
muscle building 26
myth busting 39–42, 154–5
bad foods, you need to cut out 40
carbohydrates cause you to gain fat 39
carbs after 6pm, you shouldn't eat 41
cardio every day, you must do 155
cardio will make you toned 155
cheat day theories 42
'clean diet', you can't put on fat on a 41
cook every meal, you must 40
'eat clean' to lose fat, you must 40
eating every 2–3 hours 'stokes the metabolic fire' 42

80–20 rule 41
fat loss in specific area through strength training 155
protein powder is only for bodybuilders 41
quick fixes: detoxes, 7-day slims, crash diets 42
skinny teas 42
supplements, you won't get toned without 155
weight loss is the best indicator of progress 39
weights will make you bulky 154

N

negative self-talk 265

O

omega-3 38
omelette, eggs Benedict 53

P

pancakes 56, *57*
park bench 183–6, *183*, *184*, *185*, *186*
partner-assisted chest stretch 253
PB cookie-dough bars 122, *123*
PB&J French toast 58, *59*
pesto:
pesto salmon parcels 92
roast vegetables & brazil nut pesto 79
pistachio ice cream 132, *133*
pizza, Moroccan 82, *83*
plank 163, 166, *166*, 169, 176, *176*, 187, 206, *206*, 214, *214*
plank challenge 197, *197*
plate squeeze raises superset to front plate raise 237
plateaus 261
playlist, update your 260
prawn dippers, satay 96, *97*

pre-workout supplements 38

press ups 212, *212*, *213*, 217, *217*

    bench press ups 185, *185*

    press-up challenge 196, *196*

    squat jumps superset to press ups 187

proats, ultimate chocolate 54

progress selfies 22

prone abdominal stretch 248

protein:

    fudge protein brownies 146

    gingerbread protein shake smoothie 50, *51*

    protein powder 41, 54, 146

    protein truffles 122, *123*

    whey protein 36–7

pumpkin & cauliflower curry 85

Q

quad extension 203, 227, 241

quad stretch 246

quick fixes: detoxes, 7-day slims, crash diets 42

quinoa:

    quinoa & mushroom 'risotto' 100

    salmon & quinoa bites 75

R

rainbow rice salad 114, *115*

ramen, beef 90, *91*

repetition, training and 29

reverse barbell curls 221

'risotto', quinoa & mushroom 100

roast sweet potato & egg salad 74

roast vegetables & brazil nut pesto 79

roast with sweet potato dauphinoise, the food grinder 108, *109*, 110

rowing 160

Russian twist and pass 199, *199*

Russian twists 171, 230

S

salads:

    rainbow rice salad 114, *115*

    roast sweet potato & egg salad 74

    shake-it-jar salad 72, *73*

    soy sesame chicken & cucumber salad 66, *67*

    tuna & white bean salad in little gem cups 62

salmon:

    pesto salmon parcels 92

    salmon & quinoa bites 75

satay prawn dippers 96, *97*

scapula/delt stretch 250

seated cable row 207, 235, 238

seated traps stretch 252

sets, training 29

shake-it-jar salad 72, *73*

shoulder stretch 253

shuttle runs, tag & go 201, *201*

single arm dumbbell row 219

single leg step up 183, *183*

sit-ups passing medicine ball 198, *198*

6-12-25 182

skinny teas work 42

skull crushers:

    EZ bar skull crushers 224, *224*

    skull crushers superset to hammer curls 243

smoothies 50, *51*

snacks & on the go 116–24

sofa crunches 194, *194*

sofa dips 192, *192*

sofa workout 191–4, *191*, *192*, *193*, *194* see also under individual exercise

soups:

    caramelised red onion soup 63

chicken korma soup 71

curried sweet potato & ginger soup 64

soy sesame chicken & cucumber salad 66, *67*

spicy lamb meatballs 94, 95

squat and dumbbell press 177, *177*

squat jumps 167, *167*

    squat jumps superset to press ups 187

squat press 214, *214*

squat taps 163, 165, *165*, 178, *178*

squat thrusts 163, 164, *164*, 216, *216*

stairs runs, tag & go 201, *201*

standing back stretch 249

standing dumbbell shoulder press 236

standing traps stretch 251

star jumps 171

static lunge 189, *189*

    static lunges/squats/glute 189

steak with sweet potato wedges, stuffed rolled 111

step ups 171

step ups superset to bicycle crunches 188

sticky toffee pudding 136, *137*

stiff leg barbell deadlifts 226, *226*

stiff-leg deadlifts 218, 240

stocking up 43

storecupboard 43

straight arm pull downs 219, 238

stretches 244–53

    abdominal stretch 247

    angry cat 248

    bicep stretch 252

    calf stretch 246

    chest stretch 253

    erector spine stretch 247

forearm stretch 252
glute stretch 245
groin stretch 246
hamstring stretch 245
hanging back stretch 251
hip flexor stretch 246
hip/oblique stretch 247
kneeling back stretch 249
lower body 245–7
partner-assisted chest
    stretch 253
prone abdominal stretch 248
quad stretch 246
scapula/delt stretch 250
seated traps stretch 252
shoulder stretch 253
standing back stretch 249
standing traps stretch 251
stretching cat 248
TDEE 249
tricep (and lat) stretch 252
upper body 248–53
strong not skinny, emphasis
    on 29
stronger 255–67
    extrinsic motivation 258
    fitting fitness into work and
        social life 262
    goals, checking in with your
        260
    going out 262–3
    intrinsic motivation 258
    intrinsic vs extrinsic
        motivation 258
    marginal gains 257
    motivation, keeping up 258
    negative self-talk 266
    plateaus 261
    playlist, update your 260
    tracking your progress
        267–70
    visualisation 264
    willpower vs perseverance
        256
stuffed butternut squash 98, 99

stuffed rolled steak with sweet
    potato wedges 111
success at any size 30
superfood wrap 65
superset 182
supplements 36–8, 155
    BCAAs 38
    caffeine 37
    core supplements 36
    creatine (creapure) 37
    instant oats 37
    multivitamin 38
    myths 155
    omega-3 38
    pre-workout 38
    vitamin D3 38
    whey protein 36–7
sushi, easy-peasy 70
sweet potato:
    curried sweet potato & ginger
        soup 64
    roast sweet potato & egg
        salad 74
    stuffed rolled steak with
        sweet potato wedges 111
    sweet potato brownies 129
    sweet potato frittata 147
    the food grinder roast with
        sweet potato dauphinoise
        108, 109, 110
sweet stuff, the 125–42
swimming 161

T
tabata circuits 162–81
    circuit 1 163–6, 163
        high knees 163, 163
        plank 166, 166
        squat taps 165, 165
        squat thrusts 164, 164
    circuit 2 167–70
        commando 169, 169
        laying leg raises 170, 170
        mountain climber 168, 168
        squat jumps 167, 167

circuit 3 171–3
    bent over row 172, 172, 173,
        173
    Russian twists 171
    star jumps 171
    step ups 171
circuit 4 174–7
    burpees 174, 174
    kettlebell deadlift 175, 175
    plank 176, 176
    squat and dumbbell press
        177, 177
circuit 5 178–81
    bicycle crunches 179, 179
    military press 180, 180
    squat taps 178, 178
    tuck jumps 181, 181
tart 4-ways 148–51
    beetroot, goat's cheese &
        rocket 151
    cream cheese, smoked
        salmon & spinach 149
    leek, blue cheese & bacon 148
    tomato, mozzarella & pesto
        150
TDEE (Total Daily Energy
    Expenditure) 20, 24, 25, 26,
    154, 249, 260
tempo, training 29
tofu stir-fry, marinated 88, 89
Tom 15, 16
tomatoes:
    baked tomato with kale &
        goat's cheese 48, 49
    tomato, mozzarella & pesto
        tart 150
tracking your progress 34,
    267–70
training keywords, acronyms
    and buzzwords 29
treadmill 159
tricep exercises:
    tricep (and lat) stretch 252
    tricep extensions 216, 216
    tricep kickbacks 225, 239

tricep pull-downs 225
tricep rope pull downs 233
truffles:
    avo-choc truffles 138
    protein truffles 122, *123*
tuck jumps 178, 181, *181*
tuna & white bean salad in
    little gem cups 62

U

ultimate chocolate proats 54
upper body:
    beginner workout 207–13
    stretching 248–53
upright rows 237

V

vegan burger, the best 86, *87*
visualisation 264
vitamin supplements 38

W

weight loss 23
    deficit and 25
    'good' vs 'bad' foods and 35
    myths 39, 40, 42
    realistic rate of 26
weight training myths 154
whey protein 36–7
willpower vs perseverance 256
work and social life, fitting
    fitness into 262

Z

zottman curls 221

Results

Huge props to some of the amazing people who have transformed their lives and bodies with LDNM. It is really important to us that we celebrate every success – we don't want to create an army of clones, we want You to look like You, the best version of You, and the You that feels strong in mind and body. Remember it's success at any size, and we want you to celebrate yourself every step of your journey. *Share your journey with us using #leanfitstrong.*

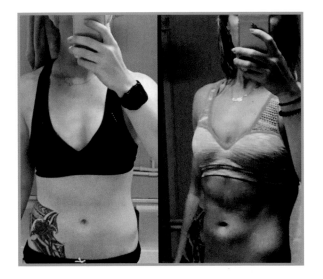
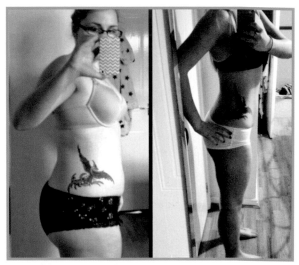

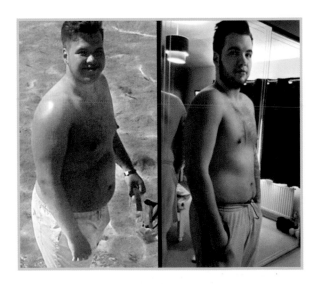
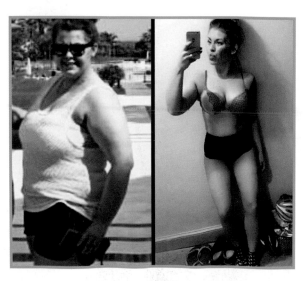

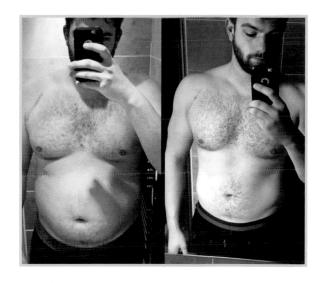
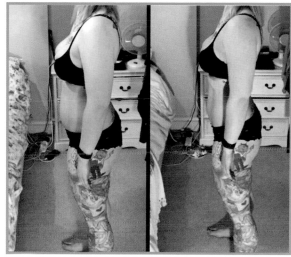
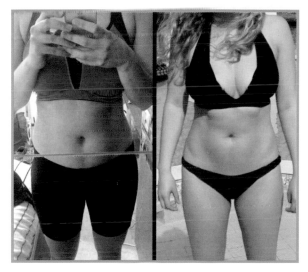
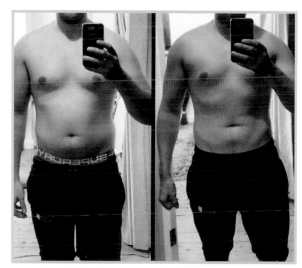
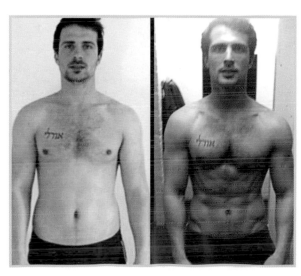
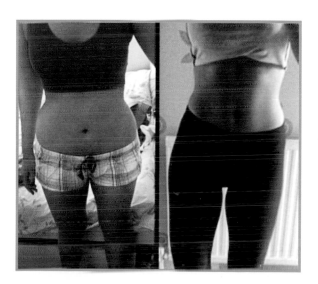

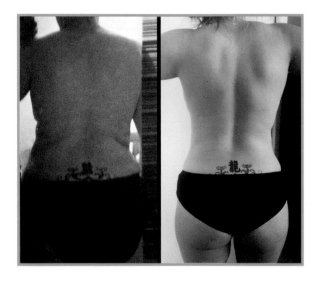
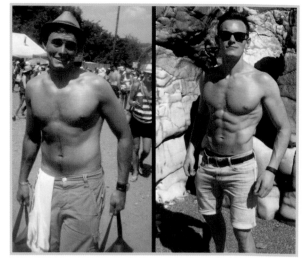
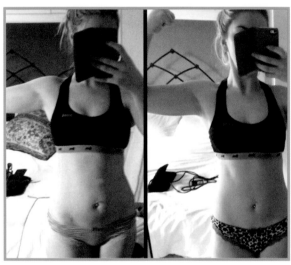
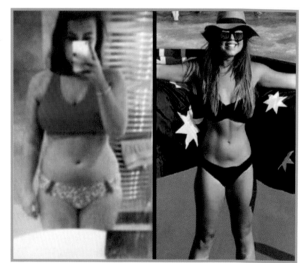
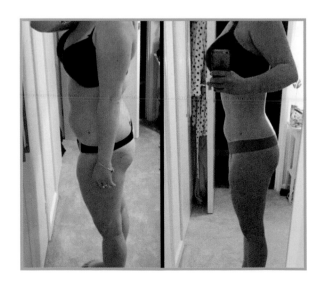
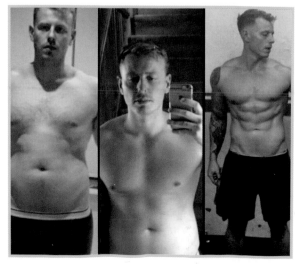

A special mention goes out to the extended members of our team; Simon Burden, Joshua Silverman, Richard Bennett, Alex Doddman (The Food Grinder), Charlotte Parsons and of course Alice Liveing. You have all been fantastic working partners, and become life-long friends.

A massive thank you to everyone at Penguin Random House and to everyone behind the scenes who helped make this book a reality: Malcolm Griffiths it was an honour to work with you, as always; Howard Shooter and Moo Jevons you made the whole food shoot the most awesome experience, your talents are second to none; Justine Taylor, thank you for your insight and support throughout the writing process; Kate Wanwimolruk and Becci Woods, your input on the recipes has been invaluable; Sophie Yamamato, thank you for your design vision, you have been a real miracle-worker; Caroline Butler and Jo Bennett, thank you for your marketing and publicity genius, you guys are amazing; and especially to our publisher and circus orchestrator in-chief, Morwenna Loughman! The book wouldn't be anywhere near the standard achieved without your hard work, expertise, perseverance and guidance.

Finally, we express our utmost gratitude to our long-suffering parents, family and friends for their unwavering support from the humble beginnings of LDNM, right up to the present day. Without your support network, none of this would have been possible.

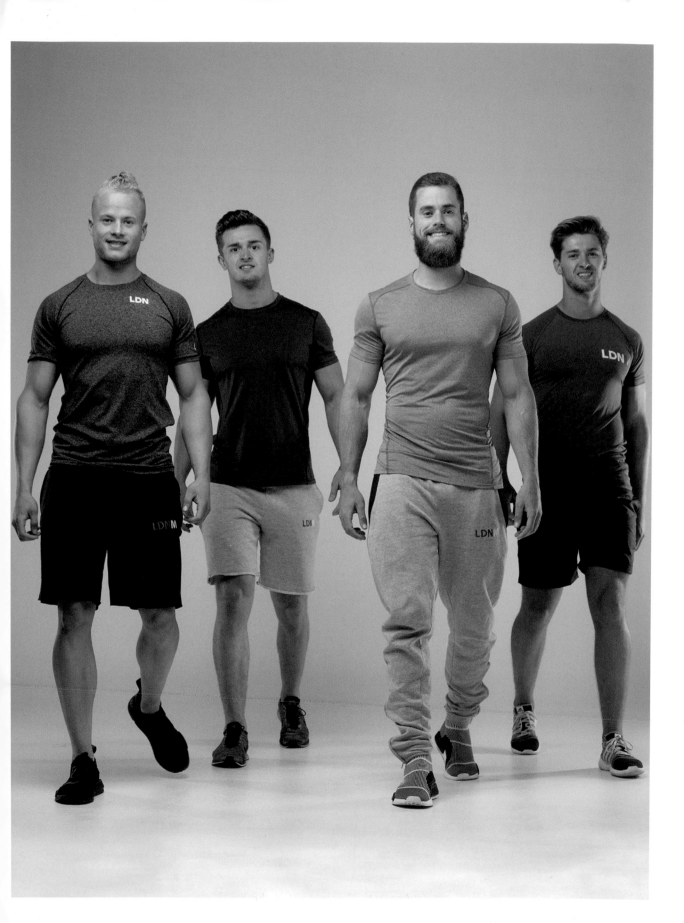

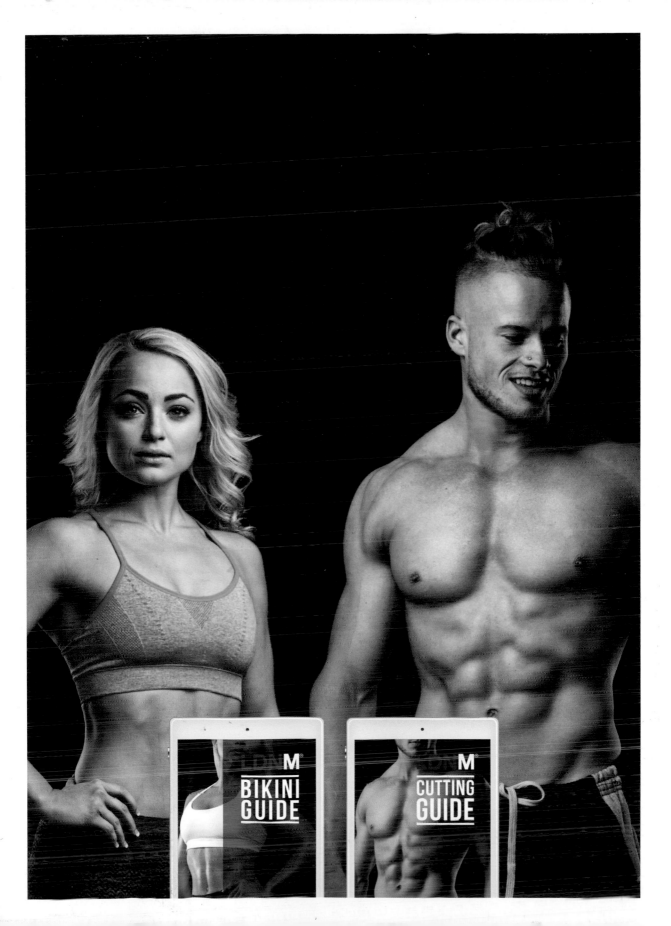